UNDERSTANDING
LUPUS

Also by Henrietta Aladjem
THE SUN IS MY ENEMY
LUPUS: HOPE THROUGH UNDERSTANDING

UNDERSTANDING LUPUS

HENRIETTA ALADJEM

CHARLES SCRIBNER'S SONS
NEW YORK

Library of Congress Cataloging in Publication Data

Aladjem, Henrietta, 1917–
Understanding lupus.

An expanded and updated version of: Lupus, hope through understanding.
1982.
Bibliography: p.
Includes index.
1. Lupus erythematosus, Systemic.   2. Medicine, Popular.   I. Aladjem,
Henrietta, 1917–   . Lupus, hope through understanding.   II. Title.
[DNLM: 1. Lupus Erythematosus, Systemic—popular works.
WR 152 A316u]
RC924.5.L85A43   1985   616.97   85-1963
ISBN 0-684-18349-8

CONTENTS

Foreword

Understanding Lupus reflects the many medical, governmental, foundation, and private enterprise circles in which Henrietta Aladjem moves from a broadly informed base with sophisticated ease. Highly regarded and respected for energetic approaches and effectiveness in educational and support endeavors for the lupus patient, her deep concerns and initiatives are well known to physicians, biomedical scientists, and a host of others at the fore of campaigns to advance health causes. As one appreciated and welcomed into research laboratories, clinics, and academic facilities as a special friend and co-worker, Henrietta Aladjem surely has identified the sites of expertise, the theatres of action, and the arenas where roles of leadership are played in multifaceted attacks on disorders of the immune system. From these vantage points, experts with unique insights and experiences have been brought together, each setting forth perceptions and projections in lucid and interesting fashion. Between the covers of this far-ranging yet comprehensive collection, the lupus patient and all concerned will find the exciting story of our understanding of systemic lupus erythematosus in transition. With the generation of new knowledge uncovering leads to shed light on mysteries of the disease, applications of research data are paving the way for development of improved methods for its diagnosis, treatment, and prevention. Here the reader will find enlightenment, and the affected are offered promise and hope.

SHELDON G. COHEN, M.D.
Director, Immunology, Allergic and Immunologic Diseases Program
National Institute of Allergy and Infectious Diseases

Acknowledgments

Understanding Lupus is for the patients and their families, for the physicians and other health care professionals and for the general reader who would like to learn more about systemic lupus erythematosus. The book is based on my own experiences with this disease, on the thousands of letters I have received from lupus patients in response to *The Sun Is My Enemy, Lupus: Hope Through Understanding, Lupus News,* and my conversations with the many physicians and psychiatrists who have made *Understanding Lupus* possible.

Understanding Lupus is the outcome of so many experiences and so much help that it is impossible to make all the proper acknowledgments. However, certain people played a large part. Dr. Peter H. Schur, Professor of Medicine, Harvard University Medical School, and Director of Lupus Research, Brigham and Women's Hospital, guided my every step and without his enthusiastic effort, I could not have completed this work. Many other individuals helped and guided me: Dr. Sheldon G. Cohen, Director of Immunology, Allergic and Immunologic Diseases Program at the National Institute of Allergy and Infectious Diseases, National Institutes of Health, has worked with me with patience and kindness. I also have special feelings for Otto Zausmer, Associate Editor Emeritus of the *Boston Globe*. Otto has spent many hours working with me, making suggestions that arise from his sound journalistic sense of organization. From Otto I have learned to be clear and straightforward. C. Michael

Curtis, Senior Editor of the *Atlantic Monthly*, has been my teacher in Creative Writing for many years. With Michael's help, I am still winning the battle against dangling participles and prepositions. I have never quite learned to manage these precise little English words.

The chapter by Drs. Anthony Fauci and Julian L. Ambrus, Jr. represent but a sampling of the exciting and rewarding original investigative studies in progress. No attempt has been made to include the entire spectrum of research in this volume.

Understanding Lupus owes a great deal to the enthusiasm of Ms. Elizabeth Rapoport, my editor at Charles Scribner's Sons, who undertook the onerous task of organizing the manuscript and putting in order the vast amount of information. I'm also grateful to all the patients who allowed me to reproduce their letters; to Barbara Feinberg, my friend and co-worker in the struggle to help the lupus patient; to Vicki Croke, my young journalist friend, who makes herself available whenever I am overwhelmed by work; and my two granddaughters Ani, seven, and Elise, five, who drove with me from Newton to Wellesley innumerable times to deliver my typing or pick it up while I waited in the car, sometimes too tired to make the effort myself.

The choice of physicians in *Understanding Lupus* has been my own. These doctors have answered questions that are often asked by patients who are concerned with the various aspects of the disease. As I have stressed, I cannot here acknowledge the many physicians who have contributed to this work, but this does not diminish my gratitude for all their help. All the physicians and health care professionals who have contributed to this volume and I share the belief that the greatest gift one can bestow on the lupus patient today is a sense of hope and better understanding of the disease. I would like to believe that we have achieved this goal.

H.A.

* * *

The following physicians and other medical professionals answered my questions concerning lupus research and the problems of the lupus patient:

Chester Alper, M.D., professor of pediatrics, Harvard University Medical School; and scientific director, Center for Blood Research, Boston, Mass.

Julian L. Ambrus, Jr., M.D., senior investigator, Laboratory of Immunoregulation, National Institute of Allergy and Infectious Diseases, National Institutes of Health, Bethesda, Md.

Stephen Balch, M.D., medical director, Jacqueline McClure Lupus Treatment Center, Atlanta, Ga.

Tamara A. Bethel, R.N., Ph.D., Newton-Wellesley Hospital; affiliate, Tufts University School of Medicine, Boston, Mass.

Emil J. Bordana, M.D., professor of medicine in the division of immunology and vice chairman of medicine, Oregon Health Science University, Portland, Ore.

Yves Borel, M.D., associate professor of pediatrics, Harvard University Medical School; director, Rheumatology Services, Children's Medical Center, Boston, Mass.

Ronald V. Carr, M.D., associate professor of medicine, department of medicine and department of microbiology, Dalhousie University, Halifax, N.S., Canada.

Lucille Carter, M.D., psychiatrist, Boston, Mass.

Sheldon G. Cohen, M.D., director, Immunology, Allergic and Immunologic Diseases Program, National Institute of Allergy and Infectious Diseases, National Institutes of Health, Bethesda, Md.

Elizabeth S. Cole, M.D., chief of dermatology, Newton-Wellesley Hospital, Newton, Mass.; assistant clinical professor of dermatology, Tufts University School of Medicine, Boston, Mass.

Anthony S. Fauci, M.D., director, National Institute of Allergy and Infectious Diseases, National Institutes of Health, Bethesda, Md.

Patricia Fraser, M.D., Harvard University Medical School, Boston, Mass.

Raquel Hicks, M.D., director, Pediatric Arthritis Center of Hawaii; associate professor of pediatrics and medicine, John A. Burns School of Medicine, University of Hawaii, Honolulu, Hawaii.

Elizabeth J. Jameson, J.D., board of directors, Lupus Foundation of America.

Stephen Kaplan, M.D., professor of medicine, Brown University Medical School; chief of rheumatology, Roger Williams General Hospital, Providence, R.I.

Richard A. Kaslow, M.D., research medical epidemiologist, National Institute of Allergy and Infectious Diseases, National Institutes of Health, Bethesda, Md.

Richard Krause, M.D., former director of the National Institute of Allergy and Infectious Diseases, National Institutes of Health, Bethesda, Md.; presently dean, Emory University School of Medicine and a Robert Woodroff professor of medicine.

Robert M. Lewis, M.D., chief of veterinarian pathology at the school of veterinary medicine, Cornell University School of Medicine, Ithaca, N.Y.

Joan Marx, psychotherapist, Brookline, Mass.

Theodore Nadelson, M.D., chief of psychiatry, Boston Veterans' Administration; clinical professor of psychiatry, Tufts University Medical School, Boston, Mass.

Madhu A. Pathak, M.D., senior associate in dermatology (biochemistry), Harvard University Medical School, Boston, Mass.

Fred Quimby, M.D., director, Laboratory Animal Resources and associate director of pathology, Cornell University School of Medicine, Ithaca, N.Y.

Dwight R. Robinson, M.D., Massachusetts General Hospital; associate professor of medicine, Harvard University Medical School.

Gerald Rodnan, M.D., professor of medicine and chief, department of rheumatology, University of Pittsburgh Medical School, Pittsburgh, Pa.

Malcolm P. Rogers, M.D., assistant professor of psychiatry, Harvard University Medical School, and assistant director of psychiatry, Brigham and Women's Hospital, Boston, Mass.

Naomi Rothfield, M.D., professor of medicine, University of Connecticut School of Medicine; director, division of rheumatic diseases, Connecticut Health Center, Farmington, Conn.

Peter H. Schur, M.D., professor of medicine, Harvard University Medical School; director of lupus research, Brigham and Women's Hospital, Boston, Mass.

Robert Schwartz, M.D., professor of medicine, Tufts University Medical School; director, cancer research, and chief of hematology, New England Medical Center, Boston, Mass.

Norman Talal, M.D., professor of medicine and microbiology and head of the division of clinical immunology, University of Texas Health Center, San Antonio, Tex.

Deborah Thomson, J.D., board of directors, Massachusetts Chapter of the Lupus Foundation of America, Inc., Boston, Mass.

Martin Tyler, M.D., D.D.S., McGill University, Montreal, P.Q., Canada.

Robert B. Zurier, M.D., professor of medicine and chief of rheumatology, University of Pennsylvania Medical School, Philadelphia, Pa.

Introduction:
An Overview of Lupus

The following overview of lupus was prepared by Peter H. Schur, M.D., professor of medicine, Harvard University Medical School, and director of lupus research, Brigham and Women's Hospital, Boston, Massachusetts.

This book was written for the people with lupus, for their families, and for the medical professionals who take care of them. It was written to improve our understanding of lupus, and, perhaps as important, to improve our understanding of the person who suffers from lupus. Readers who are also patients will gain, we hope, a better understanding of their affliction. If the reader is a physician, we hope that this book will assist him or her in being better able to recognize, diagnose, and treat people with lupus.

This introduction acquaints you with systemic lupus erythematosus (SLE)—or lupus, as it is better known—its management and treatment, and the role of the patient and his or her physician in these decisions. Later chapters go into greater detail in more specific areas.

Lupus is a chronic inflammatory disease of unknown cause that can affect virtually any part of the body. Patients with SLE also develop distinct abnormalities of the immune system; that is, in addition to making antibodies (specific substances that help destroy foreign material entering the body) against bacteria and viruses, the bodies of lupus patients make antibodies to their own cells, the so-called antinuclear antibodies. A diagnosis of SLE is likely to follow the discovery of these antinuclear antibodies, especially antibodies to DNA (deoxyribonucleic acid, the substance that governs heredity).

SYMPTOMS

Although SLE can affect any part of the body, most patients experience symptoms in only a few organs. The table below lists the frequency of certain symptoms found in patients with SLE.

Arthralgia (achy joints)	95%
Fever over 100°F (38°C)	90%
Arthritis (swollen joints)	90%
Skin rashes	74%
Anemia	71%
Kidney involvement	50%
Pleurisy	45%
Butterfly rash	42%
Photosensitivity	30%
Hair loss	27%
Raynaud's phenomenon	17%
Seizures	15%
Mouth ulcers	12%

The statistics clearly indicate that most lupus patients will not experience all the symptoms, or even many of them. For most patients, symptoms in organs that will eventually be affected are usually evident within the first year or two after diagnosis.

Most lupus patients have skin and joint involvement. We usually associate the sun with good things: life, nourishment, growth, and warmth. For lupus patients, however, the sun is more often an enemy to be avoided, because exposure to sunlight may result in a rash caused by ultraviolet rays, which can come not only from the sun, but also from artificial sources such as sun lamps, or from ultraviolet or fluorescent lights.

The rash most typical of SLE is called the butterfly rash because it appears in the shape of a butterfly across the cheeks and bridge of the nose. This characteristic rash develops in less than half of patients with lupus. Other skin areas, particularly those exposed to the sun, such as the neck, chest, and forearms, may also be involved. The rash is rarely itchy. Some patients may experience a blush and swelling, or a scaly red, slightly raised rash on both cheeks and the bridge of the nose. This may clear spontaneously, only to recur after exposure to the sun. Most rashes go away, but recurrence can result in permanent scars.

The skin may also develop ulcers, scabs, and scars or specific rashes on the skin, so-called discoid lupus. In addition, telangiectasia—abnormal dilation of the small blood vessels, which appears as red streaks in the skin—may develop, especially on the face. These streaks do not represent an active lesion.

In some patients, the skin is involved in other ways. Some may develop patchy hair loss on their scalps (alopecia); this usually grows back in most patients, either spontaneously or with treatment. Raynaud's phenomenon (in which the fingers or toes turn white or blue, with or without tingling or pain) may occur, especially on exposure to the cold. Raynaud's phenomenon also develops in patients with other connective tissue diseases, such as scleroderma or rheumatoid arthritis, and in many young or middle-aged people who do not have any associated disease at all. Patients with lupus also occasionally develop painless, or sometimes painful, ulcers in the mouth or nose.

Most lupus patients complain of aches and pains in their joints (arthralgia) at some time. Many also experience arthritis, or swollen, inflamed joints. This arthritis often affects the hands, causing the fingers and the back of the hand to swell. It can occasionally affect the elbows, wrists, hips, knees, or ankles. Other joints are rarely affected. The arthritis often lasts just a day or so in one joint before moving on to another. The arthritis rarely becomes chronic in one joint, and it rarely causes deformities. Swelling of the foot is more likely caused by fluid retention (edema) than by arthritis.

Muscle pain is a frequent complaint, and is occasionally accompanied by muscle wasting and a feeling of weakness. Bones are rarely affected, but a few people do develop wasting of part of some bones (called aseptic necrosis). If this happens, it most likely affects the hips, but occasionally also the knees, wrists, or shoulders. It occurs in about 5 to 15 percent of patients receiving chronic treatment with cortisone or similarly acting drugs. Aseptic necrosis can also occur in lupus patients who have never been on cortisone treatment, but it is less likely.

Kidney (renal) involvement develops in about 50 percent of patients. Why it develops in some patients and not in others is not clear. Furthermore, if it develops, it usually happens during the first two years of illness. Most kidney involvement causes no symptoms but can be detected by routine blood and urine tests. Although the vast majority of lupus patients with kidney involvement have mild disease and no symptoms, these abnormalities need to be treated in order to prevent permanent kidney damage or failure, which now rarely develops today. Only in that uncommon instance when the kidney function is less than 25 percent of normal will individuals become symptomatic, developing nausea, fatigue, or edema. Moreover, these symptoms often have other causes, and not all kidney disease in patients with SLE is caused by lupus.

The heart is rarely affected in lupus. However, when the heart is involved, the most common abnormality is some form of electrocardiographic (ECG, EKG) change; clinical symptoms of the heart are infrequent.

The lung is involved in about half of lupus cases. The most common symptom is inflammation of the lining of the lung, which causes fluid to accumulate between the lung and the chest wall. Sometimes this is painless and is detected by chance on a chest X ray. At other times, the fluid may cause chest pain when the patient takes a deep breath (pleurisy). This is often the first clue of the diagnosis of SLE. Sometimes a lupus patient with lung involvement develops a chronic cough. In those circumstances, however, the attending physician ought to make absolutely certain that the cough or abnormal X ray is not due to an infection.

Some SLE patients may develop gastrointestinal tract (esophagus, stomach, intestines) problems, manifested as nausea, vomiting, or abdominal pain due to inflammation of the intestines or pancreas. These symptoms can also be caused by illnesses unrelated to SLE, and they clearly warrant attention by a physician. Lupus-related diarrhea does occur, but this condition is usually due to other causes, such as infections. Blood in the stool is rare.

The liver is occasionally enlarged in SLE patients, but this is usually temporary. However, persistent liver enlargement and abnormal liver-function blood tests may be caused by a disease called lupoid hepatitis. This is a disease primarily of young women, who develop many of the symptoms of lupus (such as fever, arthritis, rashes, and pleurisy) and have positive LE cell tests (see the following section on diagnosis). Despite these similarities, lupoid hepatitis bears no other relationship to SLE, in which persistent liver abnormalities are rare.

Lymph nodes are characteristically enlarged in patients with SLE, especially in the neck. They are more likely to be enlarged in patients with active disease than in those in remission. Enlarged nodes, however, can also be caused by other conditions, of which the most common is a recent infection. An enlarged spleen is seen in many patients, again more often in those with active disease.

The neurological system, consisting of the brain, spinal cord, and peripheral nerves, is affected in about 25 percent of patients. This neurological involvement may cause behavioral disturbances, including irritability, confusion, hallucinations, and psychosis. Symptoms caused by organic brain disease may be difficult to differentiate from cortisone drug-induced psychosis or from the natural fears and anxieties any person might have when told that he or she has a chronic life-threatening illness. The cause must be accurately diagnosed, however, because the treatment for each is very different.

When organic brain disease is present, usually the lupus is active elsewhere in the body. In this case, the EEG (electroencephalogram, or brain-wave test) is likely to be abnormal, but a brain-scan test will be normal. Organic brain disease may also cause seizures or convulsions in 15 percent of patients; other symptoms, such as peripheral neuropathy (loss of sensation or very marked weakness in the arms or legs), hemiparesis (paralysis on one side of the body), or double vision (diplopia), are uncommon.

Many patients with SLE have anemia (too few red blood cells), a low white blood cell count, or a low platelet count. These conditions may cause no symptoms and simply show up in blood tests, but their recognition is important. Anemia is one of the causes of fatigue, and hemolytic anemia, a rare type of anemia, may occur in some patients. A low white blood cell count is common in patients with lupus, and it is often the first clue that SLE may be causing such symptoms as unexplained fever, arthritis, or rashes. A very low white blood cell count may predispose an individual to bacterial infections. A low platelet count may result in easy bruising or bleeding.

As noted earlier and repeated here for emphasis, most patients do not develop most of these symptoms. This list is designed to describe all the things that could go wrong, and to alert people to clues that might indicate the presence of lupus in an undiagnosed patient, or the worsening of the disease in diagnosed lupus patients.

The typical patient comes to the doctor complaining of fatigue, low-grade fevers, rashes, and achy, slightly swollen joints. Although the disease is ten times more common in women than in men, the symptoms in both sexes are the same. Diagnosis, however, is often difficult in early mild cases, especially if the patient has only a few symptoms, since lupus—often called "The Great Imitator"—may resemble so many other diseases. Frequently, patients are told only that they *might* have lupus, because they do not have enough symptoms and signs to establish the diagnosis firmly. If you have these persistent symptoms, you should be checked periodically. In such circumstances, you should consult an expert with experience in dealing with lupus patients. Patients with persistent mild symptoms rarely develop severe organ involvement. Nevertheless, the patient with suspected SLE and persistent or intermittent symptoms should be treated appropriately and with understanding.

DIAGNOSIS

How does a physician arrive at a diagnosis in the absence of specific clues? In the 1970s and 1980s, physicians in the American Rheumatism Association sought to resolve that dilemma. They surveyed a large number of lupus patients, and found eleven specific symptoms and signs that would help differentiate SLE patients from those with other conditions. To warrant a diagnosis of SLE, a patient must have four or more of the following symptoms at some time during his or her illness:

1 Butterfly rash
2 Discoid lupus
3 Photosensitivity
4 Mouth or nose ulcers
5 Arthritis

6   A positive LE cell test, repeated *false-positive* blood tests
    for syphilis (i.e., a blood test incorrectly indicating the
    presence of syphilis), or antibodies to DNA and/or anti-
    bodies to Sm
7   Profuse protein in the urine, or casts in the urine
8   Pericarditis (inflammation of the tissue around the heart)
    and/or pleurisy
9   Psychosis and/or convulsions
10 Hemolytic anemia, low white blood cell count, or low
    platelet count
11 Antinuclear antibodies

A number of laboratory tests are useful in the diagnosis of SLE,
but each has advantages and drawbacks.

The first laboratory test ever devised was the LE (lupus erythematosus) cell test. It involves taking blood from an individual, mixing
it with glass beads, and then examining the white blood cells under
a microscope. In a positive test, one sees intact white blood cells
that have ingested nuclei from damaged cells. When the test is
repeated many times, it is eventually positive in about 90 percent
of patients with SLE. Unfortunately, the LE cell test is not specific
for SLE (despite the official-sounding name). The test can also be
positive in up to 20 percent of patients with rheumatoid arthritis,
in some patients with other rheumatic conditions like Sjögren's syndrome or scleroderma, in patients with liver disease, and in persons
taking certain drugs (such as procainamide, hydralazine, and others).

In an attempt to develop a better and more specific test for SLE,
immunologists investigated the nature of the LE cell phenomenon.
Recognizing the test was dependent on antibodies to nuclei (the
control centers of the cells, which contain DNA), they used the
recently discovered method of fluorescent tagging to develop a more
direct way of detecting these antibodies to nuclei. This new technique is called the immunofluorescent antinuclear antibody (ANA)
test (also called the antinuclear factor, or ANF, test). The ANA test
is positive in virtually all patients with SLE, and it is the best diagnostic test if SLE is suspected. If the test is negative, the patient
will likely not have SLE, but the test can be positive in conditions
other than SLE, such as scleroderma, rheumatoid arthritis, infectious mononucleosis, and liver disease. However, the test tends to

be more positive—that is, have higher titers or concentrations—in patients with SLE.

Recognizing the lack of specificity of the ANA test, immunologists are developing additional tests based on the antinuclear factor that will better differentiate SLE from these other conditions. One such test takes advantage of the fact that nuclei contain many different substances. Immunologists extracted these substances from nuclei and tested them with sera (blood samples from which cells and fibrin have been removed) from patients who had positive ANA tests. They found that if a patient has antibodies to DNA or to a nuclear protein called SM (in memory of a lupus patient), he or she probably has SLE. Although of all SLE patients, only 75 percent have antibodies to double-stranded DNA and only 25 percent to Sm, the presence of these antibodies, in addition to a positive ANA test, strongly suggests the presence of SLE. However, the absence of these antibodies, in the presence of a positive ANA test, does not exclude a diagnosis of SLE.

Antibodies to another nuclear substance called NP (nuclear protein) are frequently found in patients with SLE and rheumatoid arthritis. Antibodies to single-stranded DNA (ss DNA) or heat-denatured DNA (HDNA) are found in patients with SLE, rheumatoid arthritis, and liver disease, and in persons taking the drug procainamide. Antibodies to the nuclear substance RNP (ribonucleoprotein) are also frequently found in patients with SLE, scleroderma, and rheumatoid arthritis (RA).

Some patients with symptoms of SLE, scleroderma, and polymyositis (inflammation of the muscles) have mixed connective tissue disease (MCTD), which presents a unique combination of clinical and laboratory findings. Some authorities argue that these patients have either SLE or scleroderma. Nevertheless, they have generalized arthritis, arthralgia, myositis (muscle inflammation), Raynaud's phenomenon, swollen hands, difficulty swallowing, and/or lung disease. These patients rarely have either kidney disease or brain involvement, and usually respond to cortisone-type drugs. Patients with this syndrome always have positive ANA tests and high concentrations of antibodies to RNP, but they usually do not have antibodies to DNA.

Other blood tests may be needed to help diagnose SLE. Serum complement levels are often ordered (see the following section on causes). Levels are low in most SLE patients when the disease is active. However, complement levels may decrease in other conditions as well.

Figures 1 and 2 combine many of the features of the history-taking physical examination and laboratory tests into a logical screening mechanism for lupus.

Often physicians will perform skin biopsies of both the patient's rashes and his or her normal skin. When examined under a regular microscope or a special fluorescent microscope, these biopsies can help diagnose SLE in about 75 percent of patients.

The interpretation of all these positive or negative tests, and their relationship to symptoms, is frequently difficult. A test may be positive one time and negative another time, reflecting the relative activity of the disease or other variables. When questions cannot be resolved, and doubt remains regarding a diagnosis, consult an expert in lupus. A kidney specialist (nephrologist) can diagnose renal involvement in lupus. Two routine blood and urine tests are used. The urine tests look for either protein, red cells (blood), or white blood cells (pus); the blood tests measure the concentration of either creatinine or urea. Often a biopsy of the kidney is recommended to facilitate a more accurate diagnosis and prognosis, and also as a guide to certain therapy. The biopsy permits differentiation of the type of kidney involvement. Focal nephritis is characterized by urine abnormalities but little if any significant functional abnormalities; its prognosis is good, and it generally responds well to therapy. Membranous nephritis is characterized by lots of protein in the urine, which can lead to edema. Most patients respond to therapy, but some years later may develop high blood pressure and renal failure. Diffuse proliferative nephritis is potentially a more serious condition. Many patients have only urine and some kidney functional abnormalities. However, a significant number can develop chronic renal disease or failure if not aggressively treated. Patients need to be seen often to assess their kidney function and response to therapy. The biopsy information, kidney function, and immunologic assessment often helps determine whether to treat with immunosuppressive drugs, plasmaphoresis, or steroid pulse therapy.

POSSIBLE CAUSES

We do not know what causes SLE, but the investigations being made by many physicians and scientists are getting closer to the

SCREENING QUESTIONNAIRE FOR SYSTEMIC LUPUS ERYTHEMATOSUS

NAME _____ADDRESS _____

AGE _____PHONE _____

	YES	NO
1) Have you ever had arthritis or rheumatism for more than 3 months?	☐	☐
2) Do your fingers become pale, numb, or uncomfortable in the cold?	☐	☐
3) Have you have any sores in your mouth for more than two weeks?	☐	☐
4) Have you been told that you have low blood counts (anemia, low white cell count, or low platelet count)?	☐	☐
5) Have you ever had a prominent rash on your cheeks for more than a month?	☐	☐
6) Does your skin break out after you have been in the sun (not sunburn)?	☐	☐
7) Has it ever been painful to take a deep breath for more than a few days (pleurisy)?	☐	☐
8) Have you been told that you have protein in your urine?	☐	☐
9) Have you ever had rapid loss of lots of hair?	☐	☐
10) Have you ever had a seizure, convulsion, or fit?	☐	☐

Figure 1. Screening questionnaire for systemic lupus erythematosus.

DIAGNOSIS OF SLE

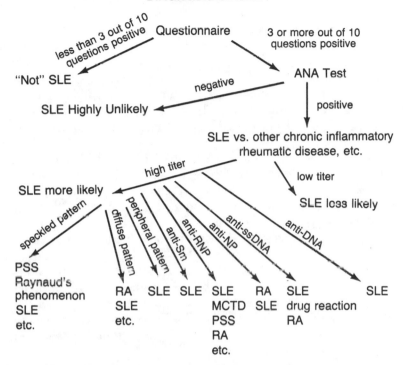

Pos. ANA test + low levels of total hemolytic complement CH50 and low levels of complement components Clq, C4 = SLE or severe rheumatoid arthritis

Pos. ANA test + low levels of the complement component C3 = SLE

SLE = Systemic Lupus Erythematosus
ANA = Antinuclear Antibody
RA = Rheumatoid Arthritis
MCTD = Mixed Connective Tissue Disease
anti-DNA = antibodies to DNA
anti-ssDNA = antibodies to single-stranded DNA
anti-NP = antibodies to nuclear protein
anti-RNP = antibodies to ribonucleoprotein
anti-Sm = antibodies to Sm nuclear protein

Figure 2. Diagnosis of SLE.

answers. Already many clues and facts point to the following hypothesis: Increasing evidence suggests that genetics plays a role in SLE and that people inherit the tendency, or predisposition, to develop SLE. One piece of evidence for this is that if one identical twin has SLE, the other twin has a very great chance of eventually developing the disease. Also, among close relatives (parents, children, siblings, and first cousins) of a lupus patient, the chance of detecting another individual with SLE is one out of twenty. In contrast, only about one in four hundred people in the United States have SLE.

Laboratory tests have shown that the tendency to have certain proteins in the blood, or on the cells in the blood, is inherited. Recent investigations indicate that some of these inherited characteristics are found much more frequently in patients with SLE. Scientists are confident that this research will ultimately lead to a test that can predict whether someone has an inherited predisposition to develop SLE.

Why does SLE develop in young people, especially in young women? Again we do not know, but recent studies of sex hormones suggest that female hormones (present also in males, but in smaller concentration) play some role. This role is being actively studied in mice who develop SLE. Clinically, however, the manifestations of SLE are the same in men and women.

What triggers an attack of SLE in a susceptible person? Again, we are not sure, but scientists have noted certain features in many patients. In some, exposure to the sun causes sudden development of a rash and then possibly other symptoms. In others an infection, perhaps a cold or a more serious infection, does not get better, and then complications ensue; these complications, in fact, may be the first signs of SLE. In still other cases, a drug taken for some illness produces the signaling symptoms. In some women, the first symptoms and signs develop during pregnancy; in others, they appear soon after delivery of their babies. Many patients cannot remember or pin down any one factor. Obviously, however, many seemingly diverse factors can trigger the onset of the disease.

Immunological investigations have also provided clues to the cause of SLE. We know that virtually all SLE patients make antibodies to their own tissues. In other words, their bodies' defense systems attack their own tissues as if they were foreign. These antibodies are not found in other persons. Some researchers have shown that this allergylike reaction is associated with a deficiency of certain cells in the blood called suppressor lymphocytes (see Chapter 3). Others have found that after certain viral infections, some animals, and even some people, develop antibodies to their own tissues. Patients with SLE often have in their blood high levels of antibodies to a number of viruses.

Given all this information, scientists now believe that SLE develops in individuals predisposed to it, and that a viral infection or similar stress can alter the delicate balance between normal immunity to foreign substances and reaction to one's own cells.

How do these antibodies cause tissue damage? Somewhere in the body they combine with antigens (substances to which the antibody reacts) as part of a defense immune reaction. Many of these antibody-antigen reactions occur in the blood, where antinuclear antibodies react with the nuclei (or nuclear substances) of the cell. Nuclei normally get into the circulation in very small amounts, but when tissue is injured this amount can increase greatly. Small amounts of antigen-antibody, or immune, complexes are generally cleared from the body's circulatory system by the liver and spleen. But if their numbers are large and the liver and spleen are overloaded or defective, these immune complexes can persist in the circulation, and may be detected by newly developed laboratory tests. These immune complexes can also be deposited in various organs, causing inflammation and damage. In the kidney, these deposits cause nephritis; in the joints, arthritis; and in the skin, rashes.

Immune complexes deposited in tissues attract a group of proteins called complement. In blood tests, this protein can be detected as activated complement or low levels of complement. Complement proteins signal white blood cells to invade the organs, which, in turn, causes more inflammation.

Because of this research, we now call SLE an immune complex disease. Understanding some of these immunological mechanisms of tissue injury has also helped develop better ways of treating patients. Measuring at regular intervals the blood levels of antibodies to DNA, complement, and immune complexes, as well as other organ function tests, often helps the physician decide which treatment might be best: steroids, plasmapheresis or immunosuppressive pulse therapy.

TREATMENT

When someone has many symptoms and signs of lupus and has positive tests for SLE, physicians have little problem making a correct diagnosis and initiating treatment. However, a more common problem occurs when a young person seeks help from the medical community for vague, seemingly unrelated symptoms of achy joints, fever, fatigue, or pains. Some doctors may think the person is neurotic. Others may try different drugs in the hope of suppressing the symptoms. Fortunately, with growing awareness of lupus, an increasing number of physicians will patiently investigate the case, performing laboratory tests until the correct diagnosis is made.

All too often, the physician is faced with the dilemma of prescribing drugs for a disease of unknown cause, trying one drug after another, hoping that one will work. Some drugs unfortunately do more harm than good, a fact that is often unrecognized. Finding a doctor who chooses and evaluates drugs carefully is often difficult.

A patient can help the doctor by being open and honest. Lupus has many facets, some of which are mysterious to the patient and some to the doctor; some symptoms may create great concern in one individual but not in another. A sense of psychological well-being comes from learning more about the illness and creating an open line of communication between the patient and the doctor. A healthy dialogue between patient and doctor results in better medical care, not only for SLE sufferers but also for anyone seeking medical treatment.

To whom should an SLE patient go for treatment? Physicians of different specialties can treat SLE patients. Some physicians specialize in the diagnosis and treatment of patients with SLE and related disorders; these are generally either rheumatologists or clinical immunologists. Most patients usually seek the help of their family doctor first, and this is often sufficient. However, when unresolved questions arise or complications develop, another opinion from a specialist may be advisable. The choice of specialist may depend on the problem. For example, you would see a nephrologist for a kidney problem or a dermatologist for a skin problem. Most often, however, a rheumatologist or clinical immunologist specializing in SLE is recommended. Referrals can be made through your family doctor, the local medical society, or the local Lupus Foundation (see Chapter 17 for addresses).

Because of better techniques for diagnosis, evaluation, and management of patients, as well as more judicious use of medications, the prognosis for SLE patients has improved dramatically in the last two decades. Twenty years ago only 40 percent of SLE patients were expected to live three years following diagnosis; now over 90 percent will survive ten years or more. Optimistically, we can extrapolate from these statistics and predict that increasingly more effective treatment will continue to improve not only life expectancy, but, more importantly, the quality of life as well.

Each patient with SLE is an individual, and the treatment (which will be discussed in Part II) must be adjusted to the problems of that person. However, a few general guidelines can be stated.

1   Regular rest is worthwhile when the disease is active, and increased physical activities are desirable when the disease is in remission or quiescent.
2   For the patient who is photosensitive, the regular use of sunscreens will help prevent rashes and exacerbations. For those who still develop rashes, treatment with local cortisone creams is very helpful.
3   Arthralgia and arthritis generally respond to aspirin or aspirinlike drugs.
4   The antimalarial drug hydroxychloroquine (Plaquenil) is often prescribed for more severe joint or skin involvement.
5   Cortisone drugs (the most commonly prescribed is prednisone) are often used for more severe organ involvement. Not everyone with SLE needs cortisone. Cortisone, particularly in higher doses, has potentially hazardous side effects.
6   If you have a fever (over 100°F), call your doctor.
7   Go to your doctor for regular checkups, usually including blood and urine tests.
8   When in doubt, ask. Call your doctor.

This book is divided into three sections. Part I discusses what lupus is, who gets it, what may cause it, and what recent research brings to bear on its causes and future cure. Part II discusses the management of lupus—methods of treatment, both ongoing and exploratory; and the roles of the various members of the health-care team: the patient, physician, psychotherapist, nurse, and dentist.

Part III addresses the issue of living with lupus. Beginning with the author's personal experience with lupus, it discusses a number of subjects of special relevance to the lupus patient, including lupus and pregnancy, lupus in children and men, and lupus in the workplace. There is a final reference section to direct you to further information on lupus, as well as a glossary of terms.

Milestones in the History of Systemic Lupus Erythematosus

Prepared by Gerald Rodnan, M.D.

Year	Author(s)	Contribution
1838	Pierre Cazenave & Henry Schedel	Credited Beitt with early recognition of lupus erythematosus (*erytheme centrifuge*)
1845	Ferdinand Van Hebra	Described in detail skin changes of lupus erythematosus under the designation *seborrhoea congestiva*: "One sees at the beginning of this illness—mainly on the face, on the cheeks and the nose in a distribution not dissimilar to a butterfly—an excessive sebaceous secretion."
1851	Pierre Cazenave	Introduced term *lupus erythemateux*
1869, 1872	Moritz Kaposi	Described systemic features of lupus erythematosus
1903	Sir William Osler	Reported two patients with systemic lupus erythematosus and involvement of the kidneys

Year	Author(s)	Contribution
1924	Emmanuel Libman & Benjamin Sacks	Described atypical verrucous endocarditis (heart valve involvement)
1935	George Baehr, Paul Klemperer & Arthur Schifrin	First comprehensive clinical and pathological description of systemic lupus erythematosus
1948	Malcolm Hargraves, Helen Richmond & Robert Morton	Discovered the LE cell phenomenon
1950	George Baehr & Louis Soffer	Treated systemic lupus erythematosus with cortisone and ACTH
1955	George Friou	Discovered the immunofluorescent ANA test
1959	Marianne Bielschowsky	Created mouse models for lupus (NZB/NZW)
1959	Helmuth Deicher, Halsted Holman & Henry Kunkel	Demonstrated anti-DNA antibody
1972	Hugh McDevitt	Established relationship of genetics, HLA, and SLE
1978	Norman Talal	Established relationship of sex hormones and SLE
1980's	multiple	Deficiency of suppressor T cells discovered; antibodies to helper and/or suppressor T cells discovered; sunscreens with PABA discovered

PART I

WHAT IS LUPUS?

This book is dedicated to Lisa Hamel* and Gina Finzi.** Perceptive, intelligent and sensitive . . . They were both in their early twenties. What do we know about their 'real' life? What do we know about lupus?

* Lisa Hamel died of lupus at the age of 23. She was an honor student in the Biology Department at Simmons College, Boston.

** Gina Finzi died of lupus at the age of 22. She was an honor student at Fairleigh Dickinson University in New Jersey where she was studying to be a medical technician.

1

Lupus
and Epidemiology

At a meeting of the National Advisory Council of the National Institute of Allergy and Infectious Diseases (NIAID), at the National Institutes of Health, I met Dr. Richard A. Kaslow, a staff member of the Epidemiology Branch of NIAID, who explained the epidemiology of lupus.

The term epidemiology comes from the combination of two Greek words—*epi*, meaning "on," and *demos*, meaning "people." Epidemiology, then, is the science of effects on people, and, more specifically, health effects on people. Epidemiologists observe, study, and, when they feel particularly bold, predict what the rates and patterns of diseases are or may be in entire populations of people. Because disease rates and patterns are determined by many factors, epidemiologists spend a lot of time attempting to identify causes and risk factors such as heredity or exposures to chemical, physical, or infectious agents. In lupus, for example, multiple factors undoubtedly interact to initiate and worsen the condition.

As explained in the introduction, several different theories are offered as to the cause(s) of lupus, and multiple factors undoubtedly interact to initiate or intensify the condition. Although a number of factors may be identified, one factor or set of factors may be important for certain patients, while another set is important for others. The disease itself may vary depending on which causal forces are operating. Drug-induced lupus, as explained in Chapter 6, is a distinctive syndrome because of the way it originates, and Dr. Kaslow stresses that if lupus can vary in its manifestations, then the medical investigators first need to agree on how to define, identify, and count the cases. The very attempt to establish the frequency of the illness in populations is, at best, tedious and difficult, even when the investigators agree on the definition of the disease.

Epidemiology usually begins with the study of such basic determinants as age, sex, and race. In lupus, those three seem to be interrelated in the way they influence its occurrence. The elderly and children are susceptible to lupus, but young adults are at considerably higher risk. More females have lupus than males in a ratio of five or six to one. However, this difference is exaggerated during the childbearing years. In that age range, perhaps nine or ten women for each man contract SLE, whereas among children under twelve years of age, the data (although sparse) suggest a ratio of two or three girls to each boy. In the older age groups, the ratio appears to decline again to about two or three women for every man with SLE.

As for race, the incidence of lupus is higher in blacks than in whites. According to Dr. Kaslow, it is about threefold higher in black females than in white females, and slightly higher still in black women of reproductive age. The influence of ethnicity may be even wider. Several studies have detected higher incidence of lupus or higher mortality from the disease in persons of Asian ethnic background. This excess risk, Dr. Kaslow believes, appears to be the case in Hawaii and possibly elsewhere in Asia as well as on the U.S. mainland. A higher frequency of lupus has also been observed in one study of Puerto Ricans in New York City, as well as among Mexican Hispanics.

Much consideration has been given to the role of major histocompatibility or HLA types, the genetic factors similar to blood types (see Chapter 2). Enough evidence now exists to make researchers confident that the HLA genes, or something close to them on the sixth human chromosome, are associated with lupus and other autoimmune diseases.

In addition to the genetic influences of the HLA system, numerous studies have been done on other familial or genetic traits in lupus. A favorite setting for investigation into the genetic origins of disease is the twin study. Such studies exist in many variations, but all generally focus on the genetic component that twins share, as distinct from the environmental influences that separate them. Dr. Kaslow believes that the significance, for lupus, of certain traits that are partially genetically determined is poorly understood. They may include such diverse features as the presence of certain types of allergy, and the level of an enzyme for drug metabolism. However, as discussed in the introduction, the study of lupus in twins may indicate a genetic factor at work.

Very little comprehensive or systematic effort has been invested in the epidemiology of lupus. Those limited population studies that have been done have not always fully used available data or applicable techniques. In the absence of promising specific hypotheses about the origins of SLE, some foundations must be laid. According to Dr. Kaslow, clinical rheumatologists and immunologists will have to be willing to work with epidemiologists to conduct basic surveys on occurrence. Incidence studies can be expected to produce clues that lead to intricate, expensive, and often multidisciplinary exploration of hypotheses. These studies will undoubtedly require financial support from the government or other sources at levels not previously attained.

"I do not want to oversell the potential of epidemiology," says Dr. Kaslow. "Many facets of lupus can be studied perfectly well with nothing other than the meticulous laboratory and clinical science now being applied by many superb investigators. Unraveling the significance of heredity and viral infection in the New Zealand mouse model of lupus does not require epidemiologic thinking or methods. Indeed, epidemiologic investigations on genetics and infection in humans will be heavily dependent on collaboration with those clinical and laboratory investigators." Dr. Kaslow believes strongly, however, that epidemiologic and biostatistical methods are absolutely necessary in a few areas: measuring rates of occurrence, assessing the contribution of certain causal co-factors, screening for disease, and evaluating preventive measures.

While much needs to be learned about lupus, and while certain epidemiologic questions are worth answering, social and political barriers may be formidable. "Whether the racial predisposition applies to African as well as American blacks is very important," Dr. Kaslow says by way of example, "but comparable data from Africa would not be easy to obtain without exorbitant cost and effort. Or, as suggested above, certain types of follow-up studies requiring co-operation of the medical community may be crucial to meaningful observations on the natural history of early immunologic derangements. Unfortunately, in this country the climate for enlisting that cooperation from practicing physicians and hospitals—to capture information from medical records, for instance—is not favorable. The resistance will be great as long as financial remuneration, malpractice, and privacy are at the surface of society's concern about the health-care system."

Dr. Kaslow says, "Epidemiology, like so many other disciplines used to study lupus, can play a role in improving our understanding of the disease and in controlling it. We must simply recognize its boundaries and obstacles. If we are clear about what epidemiology can and cannot contribute, then we can concentrate on what is possible."

2

Lupus
and Genetics

In 1953, when I was diagnosed as having lupus, I was frightened and puzzled. I had never heard the word *lupus* before, or known of anyone who had such a disease. On my own, I found out that the word *lupus* comes from the Latin and means wolf, and that *erythema* comes from the Greek, meaning "to be red." In some dictionaries, lupus is described as being invariably fatal, and in others it is defined as a generalized connective-tissue disorder, affecting mainly middle-aged women, ranging from mild to fulminating, and characterized by skin eruptions, and arthralgia. *Lupine* is defined as any of various plants of the genus *Lupinus*, Latin for wolflike, from the ancient belief that these plants destroy the soil. I found that the old English word *wikwo* means wolf and *Wiros* signifies man/wolf.

Every connotation of the word lupus—wolflike, rapacious, ravenous, wild—has frightening implications. The name itself had a frightening effect on me, and I was easily caught up in the metaphor. I began to wonder: What do I have to do with such a predator, and why do I have a disease named after a vicious animal?

I discussed this with Dr. Theodore Nadelson, chief of psychiatry at Boston Veterans' Administration Hospital, who stressed that a doctor should ask patients what the disease means for them. Patients may see themselves as victims of a predator, he said, but may also see themselves as destructive, transformed by the psychological effects of the illness into the predator that attacked them. This is not craziness, but a normal stress reaction to which everyone is subject.

My doctors told me in 1953 that I was suffering from a rare and mysterious disease that predominantly affects blue-eyed blondes with a light complexion, like mine. In 1953, lupus *was* considered invariably fatal. If the patient did not die, the physician questioned the diagnosis. Today we know that these apprehensions are unjustified. Lupus is not a rare disease. It is more prevalent than muscular dystrophy, multiple sclerosis, cystic fibrosis, rheumatic fever, pernicious anemia, Hodgkin's disease, or leukemia, and it is *not* invariably fatal.

Dr. Chester Alper, who treated me when I had active lupus, is currently scientific director of The Center for Blood Research and professor of pediatrics at Harvard University Medical School. Dr. Alper provided the following explanation of how diseases are classified, an issue of particular relevance to lupus.

"No single system of classification of human disease is useful from every point of view. There are very broad categories, such as infectious disorders, neoplasms (cancers), congenital anomalies, inherited diseases, abnormalities due to toxic exposure, and, that very large category, diseases of unknown cause. As we learn more and more, we realize that these distinctions are to some extent based on ignorance. Take, as an example, certain tumors of the lymphatic system. Some of these neoplasms may result from viral infection in genetically susceptible individuals. We also know that some congenital anomalies result from viral infection or toxic exposure of the mother during pregnancy. In some cases, diseases can be classified by organ of involvement. Pneumonia, emphysema, bronchitis, and laryngitis all clearly involve the respiratory system, and hepatitis, cirrhosis, and gallstones undeniably affect the liver-biliary tract. If we try to use such a classification, we must be aware that hepatitis, for example, can be caused by toxic, infectious or inherited means.

"Focusing on a symptom or physical sign of disease may be useful for certain diseases with a single prominent sign or symptom, but by and large, it is not a helpful basis for classification. Even with headaches, you end up classifying meningitis with migraine and lead poisoning, all of which have headache as a major or at least prominent symptom.

"The problems of classification are particularly severe when you deal with systematic or discoid lupus. It would be hard to imagine a disease with more varied clinical manifestations—and, therefore, signs and symptoms and multiple organ involvement—than lupus. Any single patient may have only mild disease, with few symptoms or signs or many different symptoms and signs—all at once, or spread out over many years. At any given moment, a group of patients in relapse might have totally different signs and symptoms, and nothing in common but the diagnosis of lupus. We also know that no single laboratory test is abnormal only among patients with lupus; the presence of antibody to double-stranded DNA comes closest to filling this role. Since virtually every organ and organ system of the body may be affected in lupus patients, it is clearly unsatisfactory to call lupus a skin disease, or a heart disease, or a lung disease, or a blood disease, even though it is all these and more. Every once in a while someone attempts to do just this. A recent reference to lupus as a form of arthritis can be particularly misleading since, although many lupus patients have arthritis symptoms of pain and inflammation, this is typically not crippling. In short, arthritis may be a minor manifestation of lupus at the bottom of a long and varied list of major symptoms, signs, and organ involvements.

"Classifications may also vary with the viewpoint and background of the medical scientists studying a specific disease. The result is not unlike the description of the elephant as reported by the blind men. For some years, lupus was called a connective-tissue disease, because biopsy sections of many organs from patients with systemic lupus showed abnormally stained microscopic appearance of the supporting tissue present throughout the body. Later, this rubric was changed to collagen-vascular. Collagen is the primary component of connective tissue, and the word *vascular* was added to stress involvement of blood vessels in lupus patients. This classification is in current use. Immunologists, however, were initially struck by the presence of apparent autoantibodies directed against normal body constituents, and have called lupus an autoimmune disorder, meaning that it involves the body's attack against its own tissues. More recently, it has become clear that the nature of the antigen (the substance that provokes the body's protective immune response) may be secondary, but that major damage to tissue in lupus may be mediated by antigen-antibody complexes irrespective of the nature of the specific antigen. Therefore, lupus is now generally referred to as an immune-complex disorder." This is discussed in detail later in this chapter.

When my disease was active, I was asked many, many times when I thought my illness began. I had difficulty answering that question objectively, since I do not know whether my tendency to illnesses in general was a symptom of, or predisposing factor to, lupus. Before the disease had been accurately diagnosed, I had developed sores after taking sulfonamides, and rashes and increased fever after taking tetracycline or penicillin, and experienced rashes and symptoms of the flu after baking in the sun. Even as a child, I had constant strep throats, recurring pneumonia, and all sorts of infections, and I have always reacted to mosquito bites. Every bite turned into a blister and every blister sizzled with pus. My sensitivity to mosquito bites and my severe reaction to the black flies in New Hampshire had led some of my doctors to suspect insect bites as a possible cause for the onset of my lupus.

Dr. Sheldon G. Cohen, director of the Immunology, Allergic and Infectious Diseases Program at the National Institute of Allergy and Infectious Diseases at the National Institutes of Health, explains that the venoms of stinging insects and the saliva of biting insects contain foreign materials that often act as an antigenic (antibody-inducing) agent injected into the body. For the same reasons that foreign biological products (e.g., horse serum antitoxins) or therapeutic agents (e.g., penicillin) can produce a spectrum of immune and sensitizing effects, so can these insect-derived materials. Dr. Cohen stresses that the allergic state resulting from insect exposure varies, depending on an individual's ability to respond to such stimuli. Accordingly, insect stings and bites can vary from localized inflammatory swellings, itching, and hives to serious generalized reactions, with shock and collapse. Since a variety of causative agents may trigger the immune response leading to production of antibodies involved in the lupus process, theoretically a constituent of insect venom or saliva might trigger or exacerbate an SLE mechanism. However, we do not now have research evidence demonstrating this to be the case. One additional important differentiating point must be kept in mind. In the case of viral infections, chemicals, and the ultraviolet rays of sunlight as presumptive causative agents of SLE, the patient is subject to repetitious if not continuous exposure. Unless insect stings and bites are multiple and repetitious, the incident is only single and limited, and the amount of antigenic (antibody-inducing) material received from the insect is small and quickly dissipated so that the stimulus is over in a very short period of time.

When I was first diagnosed, I wondered whether I had a genetic predisposition to lupus. Yet I know of no one in my family who had or has anything resembling lupus. Many of my earlier signs and symptoms had been misunderstood. In my adolescence, my mother used to attribute some of my afflictions to a delicate constitution. But my father contended that, as the only daughter, I was spoiled by my grandmother and by everyone in the family and might not have been as fragile if I had not been so protected.

The possibility of a genetic predisposition for my disease stands out in my mind. I think in simple terms: strong genes for this, weak genes for that. I fancy a series of barriers, of stages in lupus. Those with weak genes for resisting lupus would put up a weak defense at each barrier and would get the disease. In this primitive theory, it would be possible for everyone to get the disease, if the stimulus were strong enough.

In my case, infections were the beginning—the first barrier. I got too many of them, my immune system was weak, and I was treated with various drugs to help me over the trouble. The drugs, in my case, were the second barrier. Instead of helping, they caused new problems that were not interpreted correctly. My allergic reactions should have been gratefully received as a warning signal to me from nature, not just for one drug but for all. (I have expanded more on this subject in the chapter on lupus and medications.)

The next barrier, in my simple theory, has to do with stress in life. Fatigue, poor diet, too much worry—these things can erode the body's last defenses. They cannot by themselves cause you to get lupus. But once you are exhausted or lose your appetite or are overstressed or overburdened, the weaknesses of your constitution make themselves known, particularly if you are a woman. For example, the young housewife—losing sleep over her children's sicknesses, trying to balance the budget, having a cigarette and coffee for breakfast—who has some sort of predisposition to lupus, has a bad reaction to a particular medication, stays out in the sun too long, or gets an infection that is hard to throw off—or encounters some other instigating factor—may develop the disease. The early symptoms of lupus, except for the butterfly rash, are so peculiar that they draw attention away from a specific physical illness. The doctor may then treat the symptoms, and not the illness itself. As my Bulgarian doctors once said, "The doctor thinks the patient is experiencing neurosis rather than physical disease. The patient therefore goes one step further and thinks herself eccentric, inadequate, sometimes half crazy. There is no communication in this ignorance. The pills keep coming and are willingly taken. The barriers fall, the disease takes hold, and the diagnosis is easier to make."

Extensive research into lupus has shed light on many aspects of my intuitive theories about the disease. The opportunity to participate in the endeavors of the National Institute of Allergy and Infectious Diseases (NIAID) as a member of the institute's advisory council has brought me in contact with distinguished scientists working in the areas relevant to lupus. I have become aware that medical genetics is one of the fastest growing and perhaps the most commonly misunderstood area of medicine. It may be of critical interest to lupus patients. What is genetics? A brief introduction to the basics will help you understand its application to lupus.

According to Dr. Chester Alper, genetics is the study of inherited traits. The earliest genetic studies involved determining how visible characteristics, such a flower color in garden peas, or wing shape in fruit flies, are inherited. The Austrian monk Gregor Mendel, often called the father of modern genetics, observed that inheritance of such traits occurs in two main forms, dominant and recessive (Figure 3). In traits that are inherited recessively, expression occurs only if the offspring has inherited the same or a very similar gene from each parent, as, for example, blue eye-color in humans. If an individual has inherited a blue eye-color gene from one parent and a brown eye-color gene from the other parent, the person will have brown eyes. Brown eye-color is thus dominantly inherited, but blue eye-color is inherited as a recessive trait. Considerations such as these gave rise to the concept of the gene as the hereditary unit controlling visible traits. An essential milestone in the history of genetics was the recognition that the hereditary material in all living organisms is DNA, or deoxyribonucleic acid. DNA contains four simple chemical compounds called nucleotides, arranged in precise sequences, and DNA is organized into structures called chromosomes. Humans possess twenty-three pairs of chromosomes, one set from each parent, for a total of forty-six. Genes are strung out in

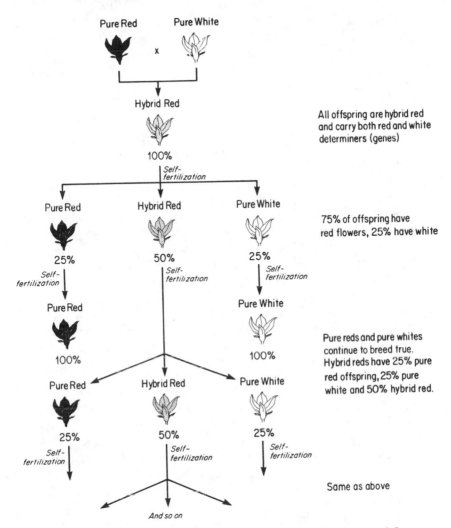

Pure Red X **Pure White**

↓

Hybrid Red

100%

All offspring are hybrid red
and carry both red and white
determiners (genes)

Self-fertilization

Pure Red — 25%
Hybrid Red — 50%
Pure White — 25%

75% of offspring have
red flowers, 25% have white

Self-fertilization

Pure Red — 100%
Pure White — 100%

Pure reds and pure whites
continue to breed true.
Hybrid reds have 25% pure
red offspring, 25% pure
white and 50% hybrid red.

Pure Red — 25%
Hybrid Red — 50%
Pure White — 25%

Self-fertilization

Same as above

And so on

Figure 3. *Gregor Mendel's experiment with the inheritance of flower color in garden peas. He began the experiment by crossing true-breeding or pure white with pure red pea plants. In successive self-fertilizations, Mendel observed segregation of the "determiners" (we would say genes) for flower color. Although hybrid red is pictured as lighter than pure red, in fact the hybrid and pure red flowers are of identical color. Thus, red color is dominant over white, and white is recessive. Only plants with two genes for white color (homozygotes) are white. If pure red flowers were darker than hybrid red (heterozygotes for red and white), we might say that white and red color were co-dominant, since both genes would be expressed in the heterozygote.*

chromosomes in a specific order. The position on a chromosome where a gene occurs is called a genetic locus (plural, loci). The possible specific set of varient genes found in the members of a given species at this locus are called alleles. For example, two alleles for flower color in Mendel's garden peas are red and white. Alleles are alternative forms of genes occurring in a given population.

An explosion in genetic understanding occurred when scientists recognized that, by and large, each gene produces a single protein. Proteins are large molecules consisting mostly of various combinations of amino-acid building blocks. Some proteins make up structural elements in cells and tissues in the body; others act as catalysts in the body's use of energy, in its building and breaking down of its constituents, and in its defense against injury and infection.

The study of genetics is closely related to the field of molecular biology. The study of molecular biology began some twenty-five or thirty years ago, as scientists working with bacteria and certain viruses made enormous progress in understanding how DNA directs the production of specific proteins, which in turn regulate the activity of the organism. Parts of DNA, researchers discovered, serve as a template for the production of messenger RNA (Figure 4). RNA (ribonucleic acid) is similar to DNA and consists of nucleotides that correspond precisely to those in DNA. Thus, the nucleotide sequence of DNA is transcribed to a specific sequence in RNA. The messenger RNA is then used to direct the synthesis of a protein (the gene product). Each specific sequence of three nucleotides codes for a specific amino acid, and amino acids (some twenty of them) are what proteins are made of. Thus the information in DNA is transcribed into RNA and then translated into proteins. (We now know that some of the DNA in humans does not code for proteins.) It has been estimated that there are 50,000 to 100,000 human genes.

Dr. Alper explained that many birth defects are caused by mistakes in a person's genetic code. Some defects detected at birth are not inherited. Cerebral palsy or certain congenital heart defects, for example, occur from accidental events during normal development and are not passed on to the affected person's offspring. Inherited disorders may or may not be detectable at birth or even while the fetus is still in the mother's uterus. The first disease shown to be the result of a mistake in the DNA coding for a protein—in this case, hemoglobin—was sickle cell anemia, which affects blacks al-

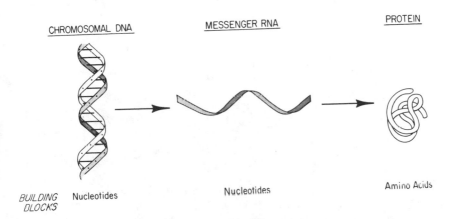

CHROMOSOMAL DNA MESSENGER RNA PROTEIN

*BUILDING
DLOCKS* Nucleotides Nucleotides Amino Acids

Figure 4. Deoxyribonucleic acid. DNA on chromosomes is organized into genes and can be "turned on" to produce proteins. The DNA has a precise sequence of nucleotides and can be transcribed as a corresponding sequence of nucleotides in messenger ribonucleic acid, or mRNA. This sequence on mRNA is then translated into a specific sequence of amino acids in a protein.

most exclusively and is associated with episodes of severe abdominal and bone pain, severe anemia, infections, and a shortened life span. Red blood cells from people with the disease become markedly deformed because the modified hemoglobin molecules at the center of these cells cannot bind correctly with oxygen. This deformation leads to all the manifestations of the disease. Sickle cell anemia is the result of a *single* amino acid difference in the 300-amino-acid sequence of human hemoglobin. This represents a change of one nucleotide in the nearly 1,000 in the DNA that code for this protein. Sickle hemoglobin is thought to have arisen by a spontaneous substitution of one DNA nucleotide for another, called a mutation, and the gene is believed to have been passed on from one generation to the next because carriers (people with one normal and one sickle hemoglobin gene, who do not actually exhibit the disease) were better able to resist malaria than people with only normal hemo-

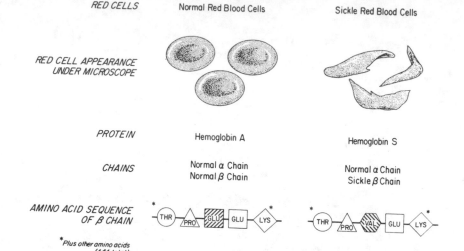

Figure 5. Sickle cell anemia, a genetic disorder affecting mostly people of African origin, is due to a single nucleotide substitution in the DNA of the gene for the β chain or subunit of globin. This substitution results in a single amino acid difference between normal hemoglobin A and sickle hemoglobin (hemoglobin S). In the sixth position of the β chain, hemoglobin A has glutamic acid (GLU) but hemoglobin S has (VAL). This seemingly slight chemical alteration produces marked changes in the solubility of the hemoglobin within the red blood cell. Under certain conditions, the hemoglobin crystalizes and markedly distorts the red blood cell so that it is rapidly destroyed, leading to anemia.

globin (Figure 5). Individuals with two sickle genes are much less common than carriers, even in populations in which the gene is common. One can detect carriers because some of their hemoglobin is normal, and some is sickle hemoglobin (the variation can be distinguished chemically), but only those with two sickle genes (only sickle hemoglobin present) get the severe disease. Therefore, at the molecular level, expression is co-dominant (that is, the normal and abnormal genes are both expressed), but the *disease* is recessive. As with all recessive diseases, one quarter of the children of two carriers will have the disease, one half will be carriers, and one quarter will be normal. Because some red blood cells in affected fetuses make sickle hemoglobin, diagnosis before birth can be accomplished by obtaining small amounts of fetal blood from the placenta. Very recently, researchers have developed methods for determining whether an unborn baby has sickle cell anemia by examining the amniotic fluid surrounding the fetus. The DNA of the fetal cells found in the fluid is tested for markers of the sickle gene. Obtaining such fluid—a process called amniocentesis—is simple and safe, particularly today, when ultrasound and other techniques can be used to define precisely the position of the fetus and placenta in the uterus.

Genetic screening may be used to test the baby's blood or urine at or shortly after birth. A case in point is the mandatory screening in several states for phenylketonuria. This disease occurs once in about 10,000 births and is a recessive disorder involving deficiency of an enzyme necessary for the metabolism of a specific amino acid. The justification for screening is that, if unrecognized and untreated early in life, phenylketonuria leads to mental retardation. A strict diet can apparently help avoid this.

I asked Dr. Alper how these things relate to lupus and what evidence there was that suggests that lupus is a genetically determined disease.

Dr. Alper answered that the evidence is largely circumstantial. Lupus is clearly not inherited in the straightforward way that eye color, flower color, or hemoglobin structure are inherited. The incidence of lupus, or some of the laboratory abnormalities that occur in lupus, appear to be increased in family members of lupus patients. We do not know if susceptibility to lupus is inherited from one or both parents.

A complicating factor in understanding how susceptibility to lupus is inherited is the phenomenon of incomplete penetrance. This is best illustrated by the study of identical twins, one of whom has disease, while the other is healthy. We know that identical twins have exactly the same genes for all traits. It must be, therefore, that for lupus and a number of other diseases like childhood diabetes, the penetrance of the susceptibility gene(s) is incomplete, and only a fraction of genetically susceptible people actually come down with the disease. This suggests that environmental events such as viral infections or drug exposure trigger disease in genetically susceptible persons. Because of the very much higher incidence of lupus in women than in men, it may be that penetrance is much higher in women, perhaps modified by sex hormones (see Chapter 4).

How does the connection between genetics and immunology relate to lupus? To answer this question, we need to understand some basic facts in these two areas that relate to the immune response, or the body's reactions to foreign or "not-self" substances. This response is complex; it has evolved over hundreds of millions of years of life on earth, and serves to protect us from bacteria, viruses, and other potentially disease-producing organisms. The actors in the drama of the immune response consist of certain cells of the body and molecules that are either on the surfaces of these cells or dissolved in the liquid portion of the blood, the plasma. In its broadest aspect, the immune response consists of a recognition phase, in which a molecule is recognized as self or not-self, and the subsequent reaction or effector phase, to recognition of an invading substance. Ordinarily, if a molecule is recognized as self, nothing further happens and there is no immune response. In lupus and in a variety of autoimmune diseases there is an apparent breakdown in this process, and there is an immune response to normal body constituents. In the ordinary immune response the triggering substance is called an antigen or immunogen. In the immune response to molecules dissolved in the blood or body fluids (soluble antigens), foreign molecules are processed by scavenger cells called macrophages that wander constantly throughout the body. Macrophages interact crucially with the main effector cells of the immune response, specialized white blood cells called lymphocytes. The lymphocytes respond in reaction to fragments of processed antigen and certain molecules produced by the macrophages that are very powerful directors of lymphocyte growth, maturation, and function. In turn, lymphocytes produce signal molecules that affect the maturation and function of macrophages and other specialized lymphocytes. The cooperation between macrophages and lymphocytes is moderated by molecules on the surfaces of both kinds of cells called HLA antigens.

HLA antigens (or, more accurately, their counterparts in mice) were discovered during studies of tissue transplantation from one individual to another. The initial studies involved skin grafts, but the same principles govern transplantation of other tissues and cells. It was found that there was great individual variation in the detailed structure of HLA antigens. This is called polymorphism (many forms) and is under genetic control like that for different forms of hemoglobin in the example given earlier. Grafts survived only if the donor and recipient of the graft had identical HLA-like molecules. In humans, the main HLA genetic loci are called HLA-A, B, C, and

DR, and the number of alternative possibilities (alleles) at each locus are many. These genetic loci are found on the sixth human chromosome, very close to one another, and form the so-called major histocompatibility complex (*histo* means tissue). It seems likely that genes controlling our ability to respond to antigens with an immune response and the strength of that response are located within the major histocompatibility complex and may be the same as HLA-DR. HLA antigens are clearly involved in the presentation of antigens by macrophages to lymphocytes and in the recognition of antigens in general by lymphocytes.

The effector phase of the immune response occurs in two main forms, an antibody response involving the production of soluble molecules capable of combining specifically with antigen and eliminating it from the body via the bloodstream, and a delayed hypersensitivity involving cellular reactions against the foreign antigen, including the killing of antigen-bearing cells. Two major types of lymphocytes, B and T cells, are key to the effector phase of the immune response. B cells manufacture antibodies. They do so regulated by two kinds of T cells, helpers and suppressors. Delayed hypersensitivity, on the other hand, involves killer or cytotoxic T cells. Recently, special means of detecting and measuring B cells, helper T cells, suppressor and cytotoxic T cells have become available for patient testing.

Antibody molecules combine with their antigen to form antigen-antibody complexes or immune complexes. Although soluble antigen-antibody complexes may be found in the circulating blood of some patients, including those with lupus, ordinarily such complexes are removed from the circulation. This happens because scavenger cells such as macrophages, found in the circulation as well as fixed in tissues such as the liver, lymph nodes, and spleen, have structures on their surfaces called receptors that combine with the antibody molecules in the immune complexes. In addition, a group of proteins called the complement system is activated by immune complexes, and some complement proteins adhere to them. In the case of soluble complexes, their removal from the circulating blood is further aided by this addition, because many body cells and tissues, including those of the kidney, have receptors for these activated complement proteins. If the antigen is on a foreign cell, activation of the complement system may result in rupture and death of the cell, a mechanism particularly useful in fighting harmful bacteria. Activation of the complement system by antigen-antibody aggregates results in the production of a number of other functions important to our bodily defenses, such as calling scavenger cells to the local site and aiding their ability to engulf and ingest soluble complexes and whole organisms or cells carrying complexes. The complement system also helps dissolve immune complexes. In the case of lupus and related diseases with autoantibodies, these processes may, instead of helping the body, result in damage to tissue. Instead of being eliminated from the body, the immune complexes continue to circulate or lodge in tissues, causing inflammation and other symptoms of lupus. The presence of circulating immune complexes and their deposition in tissues, as well as signs of activation of the complement system, serve as diagnostic aids in determining the presence of systemic lupus erythematosus.

The specific ways in which the normal immune response is altered in the patient with lupus to produce the disease is not clear, but there are a number of hints related to genetics. It is known that among lupus patients the pattern of frequency of HLA antigens is different from that in control subjects. A small minority of patients with lupus have inherited deficiency of specific complement proteins. The genes for these proteins and for HLA are part of the major histocompatibility complex, so they may serve as flags for abnormal immune response genes, or they may be directly involved in the causation of lupus. For example, complement deficiency could lead to inadequate handling of immune complexes generated during normal antigenic exposure. Recently, suggestive evidence that patients with lupus have inherited lower levels of complement receptors has been obtained, providing another possible genetic component to susceptibility to this disorder.

Since I had been hearing so much recently about recombinant DNA and genetic engineering in possible bold new approaches to genetic disorders, I could not refrain from asking Dr. Alper about them as a means of preventing lupus.

Dr. Alper smiled and suggested we discuss these things over a cup of coffee—in about five years.

3

Research
in Systemic Lupus Erythematosus

The following chapter was prepared by Anthony S. Fauci, M.D., Director, National Institute of Allergy and Infectious Diseases, and Julian L. Ambrus, Jr., M.D., Senior Investigator, Laboratory of Immunoregulation, National Institute of Allergy and Infectious Diseases, National Institutes of Health. *

AN OVERVIEW OF THE IMMUNE RESPONSE

Systemic lupus erythematosus (SLE) is an example of the immune system gone awry. Under normal circumstances, the various cells of the immune system and the substances they produce interact in a precisely choreographed fashion to protect the body from infection and other external threats. In lupus, the delicate balance essential to the immune system's proper functioning is lost. Cells become hyperactive, abnormal proteins are secreted, and harmful complexes persist.

The mysteries of SLE are the focus of intensive research, both basic and clinical. Many scientists are working to discover the nature of the underlying immune defects and are exploring possible ways

*Some of the research trends reviewed by the National Institutes of Health are amplified further in footnotes at the end of the chapter.

to repair them. Because the abnormalities in SLE are so broad, investigators are also trying to understand in greater detail how the normal immune system works. Clinical research programs are attempting to define how the disease evolves and to develop safe and effective therapies.

As was discussed in the previous chapter, key to the properly functioning immune system, in its task of distinguishing between self and not-self, are white blood cells known as B lymphocytes (B cells) and T lymphocytes (T cells). Both B cells and T cells are equipped to recognize specific foreign invaders, or antigens; when a B cell or T cell recognizes its target antigen, it becomes activated (Figure 6).

The activated B cell develops into a line of plasma cells, which produce and secrete a soluble substance known as antibody. The antibody produced by a given plasma cell line matches the antigen that activated the B cell; when the antibody encounters a sample of that specific antigen, the antibody binds to the antigen. This antigen-

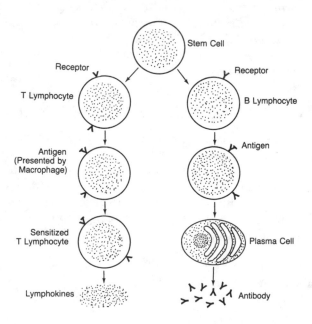

Figure 6. *The immune response: cell-mediated (left) and humoral (right)*

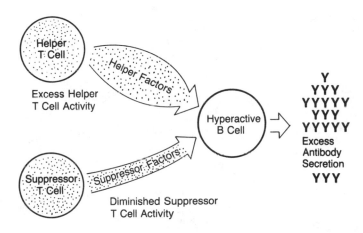

Figure 7. Disease occurs when there is a flaw in immune system regulation. Systemic lupus erythematosus, multiple sclerosis, and rheumatoid arthritis develop when suppressor T cells are underactive.

antibody complex, also known as an immune complex, is then eliminated, often with the aid of a series of serum proteins known as complement.

T cells, too, produce soluble substances; these are known as lymphokines. Working either indirectly—through messenger lymphokines—or directly, T cells perform a variety of functions, the most important of which is to control the development of B cells into antibody factories. Some T cells are equipped to kill organisms or cells they recognize as different from normal self; some, through feedback mechanisms, stimulate or suppress other subpopulations of T cells. Depending on their behavior, T cells are generally classified as either helper (inducer) or suppressor T cells; these subsets can be distinguished in part by markers on their surfaces (Figure 7). A summary of normal and excess antibody secretion appears in Figure 8.

Another type of white blood cell, the macrophage, processes antigens so they are in the correct form to be recognized by lymphocytes, particularly T cells. Macrophages can also kill various organisms, release potent enzymes that break down other substances, and secrete lymphokines that influence T-cell growth. Other white

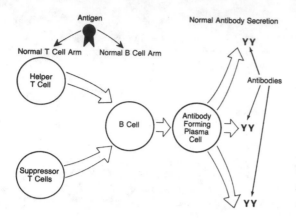

Figure 8a.
Immune Complex
Formation

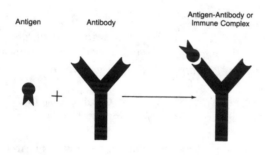

Figure 8b.
Normal Regulation of
the Immune Response

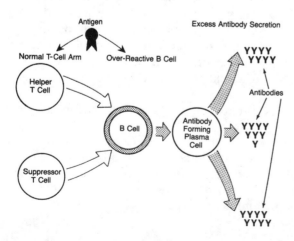

Figure 8c.
Over-Reactive B Cells
Leading to Excess
Antibody Secretion

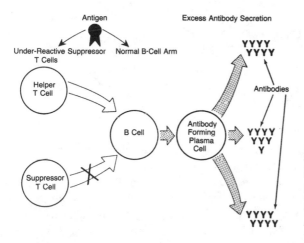

Figure 8d.
Under-Reactive
Suppressor T Cells
Leading to Excess
Antibody Secretion

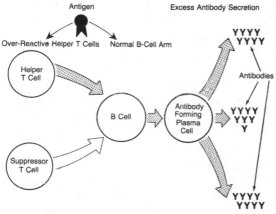

Figure 8e.
Over-Reactive Helper
T Cells Leading to Excess
Antibody Secretion

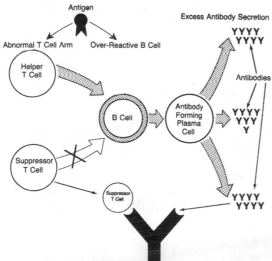

Figure 8f.
Antibody Attacking Self
Suppressor T Cell

blood cells include neutrophils, eosinophils, and basophils; these immune cells can facilitate the removal of foreign substances and release soluble messengers that attract a variety of cell types to areas of injury or invasion.

Patients with lupus exhibit abnormalities at many levels of this complex network. They characteristically produce an excessive number of antibodies. Many of these are autoantibodies, that is, antibodies directed against the body's own tissues. Most characteristic are antibodies to materials found within cells: antibodies to DNA (anti-DNA), the genetic material in the cell; antibodies to substances found within the cell nucleus (antinuclear antibodies); and, most recently discovered, antibodies to substances from the cytoplasm, which surrounds the nucleus. Lupus patients can also develop antibodies to components of the blood such as platelets, neutrophils, lymphocytes, and complement proteins, as well as to cells of the stomach, thyroid, skin, and nervous system.

The flood of antibodies produced by the lupus patient becomes incorporated, in turn, into antigen-antibody complexes of varying shapes and sizes. Many of these immune complexes, instead of being destroyed, lodge in various body tissues. There they trigger tissue damage, creating the symptoms of SLE.

Lupus patients also suffer from low levels of serum complement. Serum complement consists of a series of proteins that interact, in cascade fashion, to produce the typical signs of tissue inflammation. Some of the complement proteins form complexes that kill cells; others attract various cell types to areas of inflammation. Complement byproducts can stimulate phagocytosis (ingestion of particles) by white blood cells such as neutrophils and macrophages; prompt cells to release destructive enzymes; and facilitate the movement of inflammatory cells and immune complexes from the bloodstream into tissues.

Researchers studying lupus are faced with a host of questions. Why do lupus patients make so many antibodies, especially autoantibodies? What is the nature of the antigen(s) that stimulates autoantibody production? Why do the immune complexes accumulate where they do? And how are they linked to tissue damage? What is the role of hormones, or viruses, or sunlight? And how important is inheritance?

BASIC RESEARCH

Scientists can approach these questions in two basic ways. One is to study, in the laboratory, blood cells obtained from lupus patients. The other is to work with inbred mice that develop lupuslike disease, complete with hyperactive antibody-secreting B cells, autoantibodies, and immune complexes that lead to tissue damage.

Although both approaches provide excellent insights into the immunity of SLE, each has its drawbacks. None of the several mouse models for lupus exactly parallels human disease, so results need to be interpreted with some caution. Human studies, which require following the immunologic functions of patients over time and comparing them to normal controls, can be influenced by a variety of factors. One of these is therapy, which can affect not only the course of the disease but also the outcome of the immunologic studies. Another is patient selection: Choosing patients that fit a particular definition of SLE (and the definition of SLE is being continuously reevaluated) may create a particular subpopulation of patients, thus skewing a study's results. Patient compliance—taking or not taking medications, reporting or failing to report symptoms—always has important implications; further, normal controls must in fact be normal. Finally, because the patients being studied already have lupus, prospective studies looking at immunologic factors predisposing people to disease or causing it are almost impossible to carry out.

Blood Investigation

Many clues point to a defect in immune regulation in the development of SLE. Other people, too, make autoantibodies and form immune complexes; such structures appear to play an integral role in keeping the immune system in equilibrium. However, they are normally produced in controlled amounts. The fundamental problem in lupus seems to be that once autoantibody production is triggered, it fails to shut down.

Researchers have been studying a variety of cell types, particularly lymphocytes and macrophages, to determine if SLE can be traced to a defect in one of these cells. For example, excessive antibody production could be the result of an intrinsic defect in antibody-secreting B cells. Alternatively, it could be caused by underactive suppressor T cells, or overactive inducer T cells.

A number of investigators, including Dr. Alfred Steinberg of the National Institute of Arthritis, Diabetes, and Digestive and Kidney Diseases; Dr. Douglas Barrett of the University of Florida; and workers at the National Institute of Allergy and Infectious Diseases have found B cells from lupus patients to be hyperactive: compared to normal B cells, lupus B cells proliferate more rapidly, and they spontaneously produce more antibody. However, lupus B cells are able to respond to regulatory signals from other cells, such as lymphokines, in a fairly normal manner.

Lupus T cells, too, behave abnormally in many ways, all of which affect their ability to interact with other cell types. Dr. Ira Green at the National Institutes of Health has shown that when T cells from normal individuals are combined with serum from lupus patients, something in the lupus serum prevents the development of normal suppressor T cells. The result is that other T cells proliferate and become more destructive.

Other signs of T-cell malfunction exhibited by SLE patients include altered responses to certain skin-test antigens such as tetanus and tuberculosis. In addition, various laboratory tests of T-cell activity are abnormal.

T-cell secretions by lupus patients also appear to be abnormal. Dr. David Horowitz and his associates at the University of Southern California have shown, on one hand, that T cells from patients with SLE produce below-normal amounts of the lymphokine IL-2, also known as T-cell growth factor. On the other hand, Dr. John Hooks of the National Institutes of Health found that patients with SLE have increased levels of another T-cell lymphokine, gamma interferon (which, interestingly, is important in fighting viral infections). Both IL-2 and interferon profoundly affect the functioning of other cell types.

One possible explanation for the dereliction of suppressor T cells in lupus has been put forward by Dr. Raphael DeHoratius of Thomas Jefferson University in Philadelphia, Pennsylvania. Most SLE patients, he discovered, make antibodies that are capable of attacking and killing their own suppressor T cells. The result is a vicious cycle: unrestrained by suppressor T cells, antibodies flourish, and subsequently destroy additional suppressor T cells.

Surprisingly, Dr. DeHoratius found that these T-cell antibodies were increased not only in lupus patients, but in their families and in laboratory personnel who worked with the patients' blood. Is it possible that a transmissible agent such as a virus could be triggering these antibodies? However, another investigator who found such antibodies in patients, Dr. Peter Schur of Harvard, did not find them in their families.

The roles of B cells and T cells in the development of lupus have also been analyzed in three strains of mice, all of which develop clinically similar lupuslike diseases. In these mice, at least, lupus cannot be traced to a single immunologic deficit. Several groups of researchers, including Dr. Steinberg, have found that in one strain of mice, MRL-1, lupus symptoms seem to be the result of overactive helper T cells. In two other strains, New Zealand black and white (NZB/NZW) and BXSB mice, the fault appears to lie with defective suppressor T cells. This suggests that lupus may be several diseases— or, if a single fundamental immunologic defect does exist, it is expressed differently in genetically different populations.

Evidence incriminating a defect in B cells rather than in T cells in the development of lupus in mice has been reported by Dr. Eric Gershwin of the University of California at Davis. Dr. Gershwin found that when lupus develops, many different lines or clones of B cells become activated, at least in part independent of T-cell abnormalities. This so-called polyclonal B-cell activation produces the plethora of antibodies that goes to make up tissue-damaging immune complexes.

Still other variations have been reported by researchers at the Scripps Clinic and Research Foundation in La Jolla, California. Dr. Gerald Prudhomme and Dr. Robert Balderas, working with Dr. Frank Dixon and Dr. Argyrios Theofilophoulos, discovered that B cells in two strains of mice, BXSB and NZB/NZW, overreacted to signals from other cells. In contrast, B cells from MRL-1 mice showed no such hyperreactivity; instead, their T cells seemed to overproduce the factors that turn B cells into antibody-producing cells. (In none of these mice, however, were B cells totally independent of T-cell signals.)

Macrophages, in contrast to T cells and B cells, do not seem to play a central role in the immune imbalance of SLE; they process and present foreign antigens to T cells in a fairly normal manner

Still, certain slight changes occur. Dr. Horowitz has found that macrophages from lupus patients produce too little IL-1, a lymphokine that makes T cells responsive to IL-2 (the T-cell growth factor), and which may also help to regulate B cells. One group of researchers has noted that some patients with SLE develop antibodies to macrophages, but what if any role these antibodies play in the development of SLE is still not clear.

Natural killer cells are large lymphocytes that are thought to help rid the body of virus-infected cells and cancer cells. According to a report by Dr. Donald Kaufman from Michigan State University, natural killer cells from patients with SLE function poorly. However, the problem apparently arises at a more fundamental level, because natural killer cells can be made to behave normally by supplying them with a lymphokine secreted by normal T lymphocytes. Abnormalities of other cell types, such as neutrophils, are occasionally described, but these, too, may be due to a more primary defect occurring at the level of T cells and/or B cells.

In addition to studies focused specifically on the changes wrought in cells and tissues by SLE, more basic investigations are exploring the normal functioning of the immune system. Researchers in the Laboratory of Immunoregulation at the National Institute of Allergy and Infectious Diseases have been working out a model of how B cells become activated, divide, and mature into antibody-producing cells.

B cells can become activated in one of two ways. The first is for them to interact directly with antigen. Alternatively, they can respond to soluble substances such as lymphokines produced by T cells that have themselves been activated by antigen, either directly or in collaboration with macrophages.

The activated B cell displays on its surface a receptor for another T-cell product, B-cell growth factor, which causes the B cell both to proliferate and to develop another type of receptor. This second type of receptor recognizes yet other soluble factors, which cause the proliferating B cells to differentiate into antibody-producing cells, setting the defensive immune response in motion.

In order to obtain large quantities of these various types of soluble factors—which may someday prove valuable in treating patients with SLE—the Laboratory of Immunoregulation has turned to the new biotechnology. By fusing lymphokine-secreting T cells with "immortal" T cells obtained from patients with T-cell malignancies, these researchers have produced so-called hybridomas that secrete the T-cell products. These researchers have also developed self-perpetuating lines of T cells in culture. Once these T-cell factors have been successfully purified, it will be possible to study them in greater detail.

In work that may help to explain how patients with SLE develop antibodies to what are presumably self antigens, workers at the Laboratory of Immunoregulation are also investigating the ways that different antigens are processed and presented to T cells and B cells.

Another important area of lupus research centers on the antigen(s) that triggers disease. What is it that sets off the production of such a multiplicity of antibodies? Can a single antigen be responsible, or might a generalized defect allow antibodies to form against a variety of tissues? If that is the case, why do antibodies not develop against all tissues?

Here, too, hybridoma technology is being employed to investigate this question. By fusing B cells from SLE patients with long-lived malignant B cells, Dr. David Stollar and Dr. Robert Schwartz of Tufts University in Massachusetts were able to obtain large quantities of an antibody produced by a typical SLE cell. They then tested this antibody on a variety of antigens to see which antigens it would react with.

The SLE antibody, they found, did in fact react with a variety of antigens. These included both double-stranded or native DNA (the famous double helix), the form that occurs naturally in the cell nucleus; and single-stranded DNA, in which the strands are separated. Single-stranded DNA appears in patients with lupus, as well as some other diseases and, to a lesser extent, in persons without apparent disease.

The SLE antibody also reacted with several different structural components of DNA (polynucleotides), as well as with cardiolipin. (Cardiolipin is an antigen used in syphilis tests; antibody to cardiolipin produces the false-positive syphilis test that occurs in many lupus patients. This antibody also reacts with certain components of the coagulation system, sometimes leading to chemical abnormalities of coagulation.)

Inasmuch as all these antigens—double-stranded and single-stranded DNA, the polynucleotides, and cardiolipin—share common molecular components called phosphate groups, it is possible that these phosphate groups are the real target of the SLE antibody. These studies suggest, therefore, that the many different types of antibody reactions seen in lupus patients might be provoked by a relatively small number of antigens. For instance, a genetically altered immune cell might mistake self antigens for one of its natural targets, such as a virus or bacterium.

Still, one cannot say that a single antigen such as DNA stirs up the many manifestations of SLE. Dr. James Gilliam of the University of Texas has found that 30 percent of lupus patients have antibodies to the skin basement membrane, the delicate layer underlying the outer covering of skin. (These antibodies may represent a response to light-induced damage of the basement membrane, and may thus be linked to the SLE patient's sensitivity to sunlight.) As noted above, Dr. DeHoratius has found antibodies to suppressor T cells. And Dr. Harry Bluestein and Dr. Jerry Williams, along with Dr. Steinberg, have reported antibodies to nerve tissues in the brain and spinal cord. Although these are seen only in a minority of lupus patients, they probably play a significant role since their presence often correlates with neurologic and psychiatric symptoms.[1]

Another important avenue of basic research in SLE has been the study of factors that predispose an individual to the formation of autoantibodies. Genetic factors are at the top of the list.

Some of the most compelling evidence for a genetic component in lupus comes from studies of twins. When one of a pair of identical twins develops lupus, chances are seven in ten that the genetically identical twin will also develop the disease. Among nonidentical twins, the chances of the second twin's developing SLE are just three in one hundred.

The cells of all body tissues carry certain genetically determined characteristic antigen markers. Known as histocompatibility antigens, these cell-surface markers differ from individual to individual and are used for matching kidney and other tissue transplants. Just as blood types can be categorized as A, B, AB, or O, the cells of tissues can be categorized by their antigens, which are so specific that they will readily induce an immune response if they come in contact with an antigen-mismatched host. A discrete set of closely related antigens (they are produced by the same cluster of genes, known as the major histocompatibility complex) is found mainly on lymphocytes; these serve to regulate immune responses.

A certain few of these lymphocyte antigens are commonplace among patients with various autoimmune diseases, including lupus. These include antigens identified as HLA-B8, DR2, and DR3. At the same time, the antigens known as DR4 and DR5 are much less common in lupus patients than in the general population.

Those lupus patients who have the DR3 marker are particularly likely to make antibodies to a cytoplasmic antigen known as Ro, as well as antibodies to double-stranded DNA. They are also prone to have a type of skin disorder known as subacute cutaneous LE.[2]

It is noteworthy that persons who carry the genetic marker DR3 but who do not have clinical SLE nevertheless produce extra antibodies. Moreover, normal controls who carry this marker but are asymptomatic, like SLE patients themselves, have difficulty eliminating immune complexes from their bodies. Is it possible that these persons might also develop clinical lupus if they were exposed to the crucial triggering mechanism?

Heredity may also explain abnormalities in the complement system in lupus, since several of the complement proteins are regulated by a third set of genes located in the major histocompatibility complex. A study by Dr. Peter Schur and Dr. Douglas Fearon of Harvard demonstrated that the red blood cells of not only SLE patients but also their relatives carry a diminished number of receptors for one of the complement proteins, C3b. These receptors may also play an important role in the elimination of immune complexes from the blood.

Deficiencies of other complement proteins have also been linked to the development of an SLE-like illness. The most common is a C2 deficiency, which is strongly associated with the tissue marker DR2. However, since SLE is associated with DR2, with or without this complement deficiency, many possibilities exist: C2 deficiency may play a primary role in causing SLE; or C2 deficiency may play a secondary role—for instance, by obstructing the clearance of immune complexes; or C2 deficiency may not cause SLE at all—instead, C2 deficiency and SLE may be produced independently by adjacent genes, both defective. Researchers are attempting to sort out which of these hypotheses is correct.

Another area where heredity may influence lupus is in the production and regulation of hormones, which are known to be under genetic control. Dr. Normal Talal of the University of California, San Francisco, demonstrated that in mice the female hormones, estrogens, accelerate lupus, while male hormones, androgens, suppress it (see Chapter 4).

Subsequently, Dr. Robert Lahita and the late Dr. Henry Kunkel of the Rockefeller University in New York City found that both men and women with lupus metabolize estrogen abnormally. Furthermore, women with SLE also have a defect in the way their bodies use the male hormone, testosterone (which normally occurs in women in small amounts). Unlike men with SLE or healthy men and women, women with SLE rapidly convert testosterone into substances that can be converted to estrogen, thereby raising the level of estrogen and lowering the level of testosterone. The New York investigators then used testosteronelike drugs to treat a small number of women with SLE. The testosterone, they found, limited the severity of joint and kidney disease in these women.

Animal Models of Lupus

Working with mice, scientists have tried a number of ploys designed to alter the evolution of SLE. At the National Institutes of Health, for example, Dr. Howard Smith and Dr. Thomas Chused, in collaboration with Dr. Steinberg, have demonstrated that they can prevent mice from developing SLE by manipulating their genetic makeup. They have bred mice that possess, in addition to their usual complement of genes, an abnormal gene that prevents the mice from producing a subgroup of B cells, and typically produces immunodeficiency. When this gene is introduced into BXSB and NZB/NZW mice, it prevents them from developing their SLE-like illness; in MRL-1 mice, it curbs autoantibody production, although it does not prevent disease.

Treating mice with certain substances can also influence the development of lupus. Dr. Talal, noting that all three strains of lupus mice showed a diminished production of the lymphokine IL-2, infused mice with this T-cell product; the mice improved.

Similarly, Dr. Hugh McDevitt and his colleagues at Stanford University in California have produced remissions in lupus kidney disease by infusing NZB/NZW mice with an antibody that matches an antigen, Ia-Z, that is carried on the surface of many immune cells, and which is a requisite for the cells' correct interaction. It is possible that this antibody, by masking this recognition antigen, prevents immune cells from recognizing and thus responding to the molecule or cell that carries the antigen.

Another antibody, anti-DNA antibody, has also been used successfully to suppress kidney disease in NZB/NZW mice, according to a report by Dr. Bevra Hahn and Dr. Fanny Ebling of Washington University in St. Louis, Missouri. Again, just how this maneuver works is not clear; to the extent that DNA serves as an antigen that initiates and/or perpetuates kidney disease, an antibody to DNA might be expected to prevent the mice from recognizing the DNA and thus from developing an immunologic response to it.

It is clearly possible to modify the clinical aspects of SLE-like disease in mice by a variety of immunologic manipulations (although genetically different groups may require different types of manipulations, even when the clinical syndromes appear to be identical). However, the extent to which such manipulations might someday be helpful in the treatment of patients with SLE is not known. A maneuver that affects immune cells in the test tube is likely to have an altogether different outcome when it encounters the complexity of a living system. Similarly, results in mice cannot be directly translated to results in people.[3] (Nor can substances, such as antibodies, that are produced in mice be used in people.)

Furthermore, the mere fact that a reaction occurs does not mean that it is altering the course of disease. For instance, an antibody might bind to a cell without significantly changing the cell's function. The most that can be said at present is that these basic research studies reveal certain trends that may eventually have a clinical impact.

CLINICAL RESEARCH

In the clinical domain, numerous research programs have sharpened perceptions of the various manifestations of SLE, created promising new treatments, and improved prognosis.

Using a computer system to review data from eighteen major clinics, a group of scientists led by Dr. Eng Tan of the Scripps Clinic in California developed an up-to-date set of criteria for diagnosing lupus. The revised criteria incorporate serologic tests that have been developed since the original criteria were published in 1971, including tests for antibody to DNA and antibody to the Sm antigen, as well as the immunofluorescent antinuclear antibody test. The new criteria are expected not only to improve diagnosis, but also to make it easier to compare the results of future research programs. As was mentioned in the introduction, it has become apparent, through the work of Dr. Morris Reichlin and his associates at the Oklahoma Medical Research Foundation, that persons can have lupus without having the antinuclear antibodies that were once considered a cornerstone of diagnosis. A large group of patents, studied in great clinical and immunologic detail, showed the classic clinical signs of lupus, including skin rashes, pleurisy, arthritis, and kidney disease. They did not, however, have antibodies to materials from the cell nucleus. Instead, most of these patients produced antibodies to certain antigens in the cell cytoplasm. Two of these, which consist of particles of ribonucleic acid (similar to DNA, or deoxyribonucleic acid) coupled with protein, are known as the La antigen and the Ro antigen. Some of these patients developed antibodies to single-stranded DNA.

Moreover, these scientists were able to show that certain patterns of antibodies are often associated with characteristic clinical patterns. For example, patients with antibodies to the Ro antigen often have skin disease and vasculitis (inflammation of the blood vessels). Patients who have antibodies to both the Ro and the La antigens are more likely to have Sjögren's syndrome (dry eyes), but less likely to have kidney disease. Antibodies to a nuclear antigen known as nRNP (nuclear ribonuclear protein antigen) are also an infrequent accompaniment of kidney disease in lupus patients.

Similar parallels have been uncovered by other investigators, although different groups have sometimes reported conflicting findings. For example, Dr. Gordon Sharp and his colleagues at the University of Missouri noted that patients with antibodies to another nuclear antigen, the Sm or Smith antigen (named for a lupus patient), tend to have less severe kidney disease and central nervous system disease. In contrast, a French group led by Dr. Gabriel Richet found that patients with antibodies to the Sm antigen do indeed have kidney disease, as well as an increased likelihood of vasculitis.

In another group of patients described by Dr. Sharp, persons with antibodies to nRNP had symptoms that suggested a mix of SLE and two other conditions that involve the skin and connective tissues, scleroderma (a chronic connective tissue disease) and dermatomyositis (a chronic inflammation of the skin and muscles). For these patients the most crippling long-term problem was lung disease.

Even though different groups of researchers have reported slightly different patterns, these differences could probably be explained by variations in the way the study populations were assembled. Despite the inconsistencies, this type of clinical study helps to assess the patient's prognosis more accurately. It indicates which types of problems need to be anticipated, and it helps to provide a rational basis for an individualized program of therapy.

Another tool for improved prognosis has been developed by Dr. James Balow and Dr. Howard Austin of the National Institutes of Health. By using a detailed scoring system to scrutinize kidney biopsies, they are able to identify specific pathologic changes that provide major clues to the way lupus nephritis is likely to evolve.

Other clinical studies have identified previously unrecognized complications of lupus, including bladder dysfunction and involvement of the pancreas. The spectrum of skin lesions that may be associated with SLE has also been described in great detail. The rationale for all these studies, of course, is that better understanding of both patient and disease will lead to better treatment.

As will be discussed in detail in Part II, a major thrust of research in the 1980s is to develop therapies that combine maximal benefit with minimal risk. Although prednisone and other steroids have been a mainstay of lupus treatment, they can elicit serious side effects (see Chapter 6). The many ways that steroids play upon the immune system are under intense scrutiny. As a result, physicians are endeavoring to curtail their use.

For patients with severe and unremitting or life-threatening manifestations of lupus such as advanced renal disease or respiratory failure, steroids are extremely valuable. However, it has become clear that many of the milder expressions of the disease can be managed with nonsteroidal agents. Joint pains often respond to aspirin or other antiinflammatory agents such as naproxen (Naprosyn). Skin disease can often be controlled by avoiding the sun; if necessary, an antimalarial agent such as hydroxychloroquine (Plaquenil) can be added.

When corticosteroids are appropriate, it may be possible to curb their side effects by using them intermittently. Taking prednisone at twenty-four- or forty-eight-hour intervals, for instance, can be effective in keeping SLE under control while markedly reducing side reactions (see Chapter 6).

Another approach, known as pulse therapy (see Chapter 6), has been devised by Dr. Robert Kimberly and his associates at Cornell Medical Center. Designed for lupus patients with rapidly deteriorating kidney function, pulse therapy involves giving large doses of the steroid methylprednisolone intravenously for three days. It has succeeded in increasing kidney function and improving the patients' condition, with fewer side effects than when the drug is given orally at lower, more continuous doses.

Yet another type of treatment combines steroids with cytotoxic drugs, such as cyclophosphamide (Cytoxan; Neosan) or azathioprine (Imuran), which are usually employed in cancer therapy. Although these agents have not proved to be as effective as originally hoped, Dr. Austin and Dr. Balow have found them to be a useful addition to a regimen of daily, low-dose prednisone in a subset of patients who have a characteristic histologic pattern in kidney biopsy.

Another experimental therapy is plasmapheresis.[4] Blood is withdrawn from the patient, and the patient's blood cells are separated from the plasma, the liquid part of the blood. The plasma, containing antibodies and immune complexes, is discarded; blood cells are returned to the patient, along with an albumin solution to replace the discarded plasma.

Plasmapheresis clearly succeeds in lowering the level of circulating immune complexes, which initiate much of the tissue damage in SLE. Other potentially beneficial effects of the process include unclogging the immune system's disposal mechanisms and removing factors that affect various cellular functions. Despite certain risks— including the removal or replacement of too much fluid, infection, or bleeding problems caused by the removal of clotting factors— plasmapheresis has benefited some patients with lupus.

Dr. John Verrie Jones and his colleagues at Chicago's Rush-Presbyterian Medical Center have used plasmapheresis in combination with prednisone and a cytotoxic agent to treat patients known to have high levels of circulating immune complexes. Following plasmapheresis, these patients experienced improvements in neurologic function, kidney disease, and crippling arthritis. Similarly, at the National Institutes of Health plasmapheresis has been used to treat a subgroup of patients with high levels of circulating immune complexes, antibodies to the Ro antigen, and severe vasculitis, including life-threatening bowel vasculitis. These patients responded to plasmapheresis combined with prednisone and a cytotoxic agent, whereas they had failed to respond to prednisone and the cytotoxic agent alone. A coordinated study evaluating the short-term and long-term effectiveness and the risks of plasmapheresis in patients with severe forms of lupus nephritis is now under way at fourteen institutions around the country.

Ameliorating the complications of lupus is the goal of other new forms of therapy. All patients taking corticosteroids, including SLE patients, are prone to develop problems with blood supply to certain bones, which can lead to death of bony tissues. Dr. Thomas Zizic and his associates at Johns Hopkins University have developed sensitive tests to detect this condition and have demonstrated that it is possible to prevent bone destruction from occurring by surgery to relieve the pressure in the affected bones.

Many groups have tried to find ways to manage the dry eyes that can accompany SLE, sometimes causing permanent visual damage. Dr. Robert Fox and his co-workers at Scripps have found that some patients do well when eye drops consisting of the patient's own serum diluted with saline are applied at frequent intervals.

In addition to the therapies currently being evaluated in clinical situations,[5] many basic research projects may eventually yield new forms of treatment. For example, the anti-DNA antibodies and the anti-Ia antibodies that reverse lupus kidney disease in mice may someday prove useful in people as well. Substances produced by immune cells, like the lymphokine IL-2, may also help to alleviate human lupus. Alternatively, better chemotherapeutic agents may make it possible to target specific cell populations. Perhaps even antiviral agents may be called into play.

For the present, however, these all remain a matter of speculation. In the years ahead, as research continues to peel away one layer after another of the complexity that surrounds immunity and lupus, these possibilities must be submitted to testing, first in the laboratory and then in controlled clinical trials. Some of the research trends reviewed by the National Institutes of Health are amplified in the notes that follow:

*   *   *

[1] Dr. Ronald V. Carr, associate professor, department of medicine and department of microbiology, Dalhousie University, Halifax, Nova Scotia, Canada, has conducted research suggesting that ingested antigens could play a role in pathogenesis of systemic lupus erythematosus. His major scientific interest is the role of immune complexes in diseases and regulation of mucosal immunity. (Mucosa is the term used to describe the tissue lining the mouth, nose, respiratory tract, digestive tract, and other sites where the inside of the body comes in contact with the outside environment.) Dr. Carr is also very interested in the possibility that food antigens play a role in the development of autoimmune diseases. Although a group at the National Institutes of Health lead by Dr. Alfred Steinberg has been doing similar studies, Dr. Carr's research is unique.

Dr. Carr and his colleagues discovered that sera from certain SLE patients contained antibodies to BGG (bovine gamma globulin) and BSA (bovine serum albumin), presumably as a consequence of the ingestion of milk and beef, which contain these substances.

I listened to Dr. Carr with strangely mixed feelings. I remembered my own difficulties with milk and my aversion to beef. When I eat beef or drink milk, I develop the same discomfort I do when I stay out in the sun or take certain medication. I recalled the time when I had active lupus and was tested for an intolerance to milk. My doctor explained to me that lactose, or milk sugar, could not be taken up directly by the intestine. It first had to be broken down by an enzyme called lactase into two simple sugars—glucose and galactose. These smaller molecules could be absorbed more easily. The test showed that after taking lactose sugar I had no elevation of my blood glucose, the normal sugar of the blood, which would be expected if the lactose had been broken down. On the other hand, I tolerated a mixture of glucose and galactose without stress. This indicated that I could not digest milk properly. Now I wondered if my intolerance to milk was more complicated. Dr. Carr is investigating whether the sort of discomfort some lupus patients feel when they consume beef and milk is related to the presence of the BGG and BSA antibodies.

Dr. Carr's studies are not directed at nutrition per se for people with SLE but at the possibility that some of the abnormalities seen in SLE are a result of an immunologic reaction to food antigens. That is, on exposure to certain foods, patients with SLE may absorb food material into the bloodstream that will react with antibodies directed against these foods. The resultant immune complexes might then circulate, become trapped in certain tissues like the skin or kidneys, and cause an inflammatory reaction. This, in turn, could damage the organ, and perhaps lead to a rash in the skin or nephritis in the kidney. Lupus patients are known to have more antibodies to certain milk proteins than most people. Studies also have shown that related food antigens such as BGG and casein, a protein in cow's milk, do enter the circulation; in some patients, researchers have found these substances, and specific antibodies to them, in the blood simultaneously, leading them to suspect that immune complexes of these foods can and do form. However, Dr. Carr stresses that they have not yet demonstrated immune complexes containing food antigens in the kidneys or skin of lupus patients.

Dr. Carr's interest in the possibility that food contains immune complexes came about accidentally. He had actually been studying DNA, looking for DNA antibodies, when he discovered that the sera were reacting with BGG, as well as with milk and beef extract, both of which contained BGG. Since these two foods are staples in the diet, and thus are consumed daily in some form or another, Dr. Carr's research team began their comprehensive study of the possibility that food can play a role in immune complex formation.

This fortuitous finding exhibits, in a way, one of my favorite definitions of research, which is from Albert Szyent-Georgy: "To see what everyone has seen, and think what no one else has thought."

Furthermore, for a number of years we have known that people who have an IgA deficiency (a decrease or lack of the main antibody found in the digestive tract and other mucosal areas) have increased levels of antibodies to milk proteins. Of considerable interest is that people with IgA deficiency also have an increased frequency of autoimmune diseases. We also know that IgA tends to inhibit absorption of immunologically active food from the digestive tract. This information led Dr. Robert Good, then at the University of Minnesota, to suggest that the higher incidence of autoimmunity in IgA-deficient people might be explained by the increased amount of absorbed food antigens (which might cross-react with the individual's own tissue components, which would stimulate an autoimmune response. (A cross-reaction means that two different substances have certain similar features, and an antibody against one will react with the other because of the similar features.) Since food is clearly loaded with animal or vegetable tissues and tissue components, Dr. Good theorized that absorption of these "foreign" materials might trigger an autoimmune response. Furthermore, the prevalence of IgA deficiency is increased from the general population frequency of about 1:700, to 1:25 in lupus. Although this is a relatively small proportion of SLE patients (4 percent), it may be a clue in the search for factors important in the development of some cases of lupus.

Another very closely related area of Dr. Carr's work stems from the recent discovery that certain T lymphocytes play a major role in the regulation of antibody formation. One subset of these T cells is called T suppressor cells because they can suppress, or turn down, the immune response. Current evidence indicates that one of the basic problems in SLE may be a defect in the function of these T suppressor cells. Recently, Dr. Carr and other researchers have found that the normal immune response to food is stimulation of the local production of IgA antibodies, and a specific suppression of the systemic response of IgG (and IgM) antibodies to the food substance, a suppression that often appears to be due to T suppressor cells. IgG and IgM antibodies are the 2 major antibody classes of the systemic (as opposed to the mucosal) immune system.

An exciting new development in this area is Dr. Carr's finding that NZB/NZW mice (a strain of mice that develop a disease very much like human SLE) fail to show this normal suppressive sequence when fed BGG, and actually show an eightfold increase in antibody to BGG when subsequently immunized. "This finding," said Dr. Carr, "has potentially great significance in helping us to understand SLE. We already know that foreign proteins which cross-react with "self" proteins can cause disease if an immune response occurs. For example, if foreign thyroglobulin (one of the proteins of the thyroid gland) is injected into rabbits, an autoimmune inflammation of the thyroid gland can develop, because the rabbit makes antibodies to the foreign thyroglobulin, which results in the formation of cross-reacting autoantibodies that attack the similarly structured rabbit thyroglobulin. Oral tolerance induction (the term used to denote the suppressive sequence described above) might be a protective mechanism in normal animals, which helps to prevent autoimmune phenomena analogous to the rabbit thyroiditis (thyroid inflammation) triggered by food-antigen exposure. The development of oral tolerance would help to prevent the animal from mounting massive immune responses against such food antigens, many of which would clearly be similar to many 'self' antigens. The failure of oral tolerance in NZB/NZW mice might therefore lead to some of the autoimmune problems seen in these animals. By inference, a similar failure in SLE could account for the high levels of antibodies to BGG and casein that have been found."

In recent studies Dr. Carr has found that although the NZB/NZW mice react abnormally to BGG, they do tolerate egg-white albumin. This is of great interest, since he has also found that SLE patients have normal levels of antibody to this protein. Thus the way the mice respond to these food substances seems to parallel the way that SLE patients react to them, and considerably strengthens the possibility that by studying the mice Dr. Carr will be able to unravel the response to food in lupus patients. Dr. Carr's group is now studying the response of the NZB/NZW mice to casein, a protein in cow's milk to which SLE patients have very high levels of antibody. Preliminary results indicate that the mice do not tolerate to casein normally either. The research team led by Dr. Alfred Steinberg of NIH has also found variations in mice's ability to tolerate with different food antigens, depending on the autoimmune mouse strain being studied. These variations may correspond to those seen in different lupus patients.

According to Dr. Carr, the inability of lupus patients to tolerate certain foods might contribute to the disease development, either by food antigen containing immune complexes, or the development of autoantibodies secondary to the cross-reacting food stimulus. Furthermore, suppressor T cells are apparently activated by exposure to immune complexes that contain antibodies of specific classes, and the suppressor cells that decrease the specific systemic immune response after ingestion of food apparently come from the region of the intestinal tract where IgA is the predominant antibody. There is therefore the possibility of an intriguing connection between IgA deficiency, food reactivity, and autoimmune diseases like SLE.

Dr. Carr hypothesizes that in IgA-deficient individuals, the suppressor cells that are normally activated in the region of the intestine by immune complexes containing IgA antibodies (the intestinal antibodies) and by food might never be triggered, because there is little or no IgA. Thus, no suppression of the systemic immune system occurs. In addition, absorption of the food into the bloodstream might occur more rapidly because of the lack of IgA. (Other researchers have shown that IgA decreases absorption of immunologically active food.) This combination of failure of suppression and increased circulating antigen may lead to an increased systemic immune response, which could result in the formation of damaging immune complexes and/or autoantibodies.

Dr. Carr cautioned that this is purely a hypothesis. He and his colleagues are intensively examining various aspects of this theory, because it will help them understand the integration of immune regulation in the different systems of the body and may directly point to certain pathogenic factors in at least some patients with SLE. Dr. Carr also pointed out that, as with many things, the IgA theory has two sides. Some patients with SLE and other diseases have IgA deposits in their kidneys. Researchers are attempting to determine if these deposits contain food antigens. "In this case, rather than failing to produce systemic suppression, the cell defects may actually result in an increase in IgA antibody to food," said Dr. Carr, "and immune complexes (containing the food in question and the specific IgA antibody) may deposit, leading to tissue damage. Such a mechanism may occur in some cases of a disease called anaphylactoid purpura, especially in children. In this disease, symptoms often include nephritis, a rash, and digestive tract disturbances. IgA deposits, which look like immune complex deposits, are often found in the kidney and the skin, and we have found a very high prevalence of antibodies to both casein and BGG, as well as circulating antigen and immune complexes, in the sera of these patients. We are now working to show whether food antigens and antibodies are in the immune deposits in their tissues."

The research of another investigative team also seems to implicate ingested antigens as a possible trigger for lupus. Recently Dr. Emil J. Bordana and his colleagues reported that a diet high in alfalfa sprouts produced a lupuslike syndrome in some macaque monkeys.

Dr. Bordana is professor of medicine in the division of immunology and current vice chairman of medicine at Oregon Health Science University, Portland, Oregon. The importance of his research and observations is that his laboratory has induced a lupuslike syndrome in a primate using an ingested material common to many of the legumes. This has repercussions with respect to this and similar substances that are consumed by the public on a daily basis.

Dr. Bordana's project began with recent observations made with his collaborator, Dr. M. Rene Malinow of the Oregon Regional Primate Research Center, that both germinated and ungerminated alfalfa seed caused the development of a lupuslike illness in female macaque monkeys. The alfalfa seed was originally being tested to see if it would lower plasma cholesterol, and it had displayed remarkable potential in both rabbits and monkeys. This was Dr. Malinow's original research interest, and in order to explore whether the seed acted to improve plasma cholesterol in humans, Dr. Malinow began to consume some himself. Aside from noting a striking reduction of his plasma cholesterol, he noted development of lupuslike symptoms of mild anemia, thrombocytopenia (reduction of platelets), and leukopenia (lowered leukocyte levels in the blood), along with the development of antinuclear antibodies, which promptly normalized on cessation of alfalfa seed ingestion. It was this observation, published in *Lancet* (1:615, 1981), that prompted studies in monkeys that had been fed alfalfa seed.

The original study group consisted of ten female macaques, five of whom were fed a semipurified diet known to be nourishing and without harmful effects. The remaining five were given the same diet with the addition of 45 percent ground alfalfa seed. Those animals not exposed to alfalfa seed remained entirely well and developed no physical or laboratory signs of systemic lupus erythematosus. However, three of the five monkeys ingesting the alfalfa seed became ill. One monkey had all the clinical and serologic findings characterizing spontaneous systemic lupus erythematosus in humans. A mild facial rash was evident with loss of hair. This also included development of antiglobulin-positive hemolytic anemia, high titer of antinuclear antibodies, lowered complement proteins, and remarkable amounts of antinative DNA antibody. Both skin and kidney biopsies indicated the presence of inflammatory changes identical to patterns of lupus encountered in humans. The other two monkeys became ill in a similar fashion. One quickly died of infection. The other, though it developed anemia, autoantibodies, a mild rash, and alopecia, did not develop nephritis on biopsy. Both animals who became ill and survived were taken off alfalfa seed.

Despite this, the illness persisted and later responded dramatically to a short treatment with corticosteroids. Addition of seeds to their diet led to an immediate flare of symptoms. Based on these observations, it was hypothesized that alfalfa seed contained a material that triggered the onset of disease in susceptible monkeys. These preliminary observations were published in the *American Journal of Kidney Disease* (1:345–352, 1982).

A second preliminary study was carried out in a group of twelve female macaques. Dr. Malinow and Dr. Bordana wished to explore the possibility that germinated alfalfa seed (sprouts) might also cause development of illness. In addition, they began to suspect that L-canavanine, a nonprotein amino acid and structural analogue of arginine (an amino acid that is an essential component of many proteins), might be the offending culprit in alfalfa seed. Six animals (so-called control monkeys) were fed a semipurified diet, and the remaining six were fed similar food containing 40 percent overdried alfalfa sprouts. Each of the control animals and four of the six monkeys ingesting alfalfa sprouts did not show abnormalities during the period of observation, with the exception that one monkey fed sprouts developed a significant titer of antinuclear antibody. However, the other two animals developed significant hemolytic anemia with antinuclear antibody, antibody to DNA, and lowered complement levels. One animal died of infections and the other completely recovered after being taken off alfalfa sprouts and returned to its regular diet.

Two additional monkeys in which SLE had developed after ingestion of alfalfa seed were normal after being fed their regular diet for a year. These two monkeys, as well as the sprout survivor above, were fed 1 percent L-canavanine sulfate in a semipurified diet. After one to two months of observation, each of the three monkeys became anemic, and two developed antinuclear antibodies, slight elevations of antibody to DNA, and lowered serum complement. The animals recovered after return to a normal diet.

These preliminary data suggest that alfalfa sprouts induce an SLE-like syndrome similar to that noted in monkeys ingesting alfalfa seed. Since not all animals are equally susceptible, a genetically modulated mechanism might be operative. As well, Dr. Malinow and Dr. Bordana's findings suggest that L-canavanine—which occurs naturally in relatively large concentrations in alfalfa seeds and sprouts—may be involved, since this amino acid reactivates SLE in monkeys.

L-canavanine may substitute for arginine in proteins that control the function of DNA. These observations and their significance were recently reported in *Science* (216:415–417, 1982).

The capacity to reproduce SLE in nonhuman primates is unprecedented and will offer a unique model for future studies relating to genetic, hormonal, or dietary factors operative in the development of this disease. A monkey model for lupus would also permit more pertinent studies relating to the causative mechanisms involved in the disease, along with innovative modalities of treatment.*

Recent observations indicate that sera from patients with SLE contain antibodies to alfalfa seed extract. Similar antibodies were not seen in sera from normal individuals or patients with non-SLE rheumatic disorders. The antibody to alfalfa seed extract reacts in a similar way immunologically as antibody directed against native DNA. The immunogenic agent in alfalfa seed seems to be present in native DNA. This shared antigen may be L-canavanine (*Journal of Allergy and Clinical Immunology* 71:102, 1983).

Subsequent studies have been carried out to remove L-canavanine content from alfalfa seed by autoclaving, a process that uses high temperature and pressure. L-canavanine was undetectable after three hours of autoclaving. This ground, autoclaved alfalfa seed, incorporated at the 45 percent level in a semipurified diet containing cholesterol, was given to eleven monkeys for one year. A second group of seventeen control monkeys were maintained on a similar diet lacking alfalfa seed. Periodic blood, serological, and complement studies were carried out in all animals. No evidence of an SLE-like syndrome was observed in either group of animals. However, the average plasma cholesterol levels of the monkeys fed the autoclaved alfalfa seed were lower than that of the second group. Thus, autoclaved alfalfa seed prevents elevated cholesterol levels without signs of an SLE-like syndrome in monkeys. These results may be useful in treating humans with high cholesterol levels (*Federation Proceedings of the American Societies of Experimental Biology*, **42**:1056, 1983).

* * *

[2] Dr. Ronald V. Carr and his colleagues at Dalhousie University are among the researchers investigating the possibility that there may

* This research is partially supported by the Lupus Foundation of America, Inc.

be something transmissible in lupus, although the disease is not infectious in the usual sense. While studying DNA antibodies in SLE patients, Dr. Carr's research team found a number of normal individuals who have significant elevations of antibodies to single-stranded DNA. Lupus patients can have antibodies to either single-stranded or double-stranded DNA, but antibodies to single-stranded DNA are much more common. Research has shown that most normal people with elevated antibodies to single-stranded DNA had worked in laboratories studying SLE! In fact, about one third of the people working in SLE labs have this increase. Dr. Carr's colleagues wondered if this was due to a transmissible stimulus, and why it afflicted only one third of the SLE lab workers, since they could not relate it to age, sex, duration of working in the laboratory, or any of a number of other factors.

Studies done by a host of others in mice and, more recently, in humans reveal that certain genetic factors play a major role in immune regulation, and also appear to play a role in human diseases associated with the immune system. For example, over 90 percent of patients with ankylosing spondylitis, a rheumatic disease, have a genetic factor called HLA-B27. Toward the end of 1978, two groups, one at the National Institutes of Health and one at Rockefeller University in New York, found that 70 to 80 percent of lupus patients have two genetic antigens, one called DR2 and another called DR3. This combination occurs in almost one third of the general population, the same proportion Dr. Carr found among the laboratory workers who showed an increase in antibodies to single-stranded DNA (anti-DNA). Dr. Carr's next step will be to examine the genetic types of the laboratory people, especially since another research team has recently found that DR3 alone appears to be associated with anti-DNA in SLE and other diseases. If Dr. Carr's researchers find that the one third who are reacting have a very high frequency of both DR2 and DR3, that will strongly support the concept that regulation of the ability to form significantly elevated levels of antibodies to DNA might be associated with these or closely related genetic factors. It might also support the idea that, in humans, certain genetic factors involved in the control of immune regulation play a major role in the development of autoantibodies, and thus perhaps in the onset of autoimmune diseases. If true, this hypothesis should contribute to the understanding of the factors involved in the development of SLE.

Further support for the role of an environmental factor, if not a transmissible one, comes from the work of Dr. R. DeHoratius and Dr. R. Messner of the University of Minnesota, who found elevated levels of antilymphocyte antibodies in household contacts of SLE patients, whether they were blood relatives or not. Other changes in contacts have been reported by Dr. Naomi Rothfield of the University of Connecticut School of Medicine. It is very important to stress that none of these investigators believe that their studies indicate that lupus is infectious, and thus patients' relatives and friends should not be afraid of ever "catching" it.

* * *

[3] Mice and macaque monkeys are not the only creatures used as animal models for lupus. Dr. Robert Schwartz is professor of medicine at Tufts University Medical School, and director of cancer research, chief of hematology, New England Medical Center. Dr. Schwartz told me that once he came across a lupus patient with every single symptom of the disease—a female white poodle. Dr. Robert M. Lewis, from Laboratory Animal Resources, Cornell University School of Medicine, was puzzled by the dog's symptoms, and had brought her to Dr. Schwartz's attention. Together they made a diagnosis of lupus.

Since they diagnosed that first dog, Dr. Schwartz and Dr. Lewis have seen many more dogs with lupus, and have found that the canine version of lupus erythematosus is strikingly similar to human systemic lupus erythematosus. It includes positive lupus erythematosus cell tests, antibodies to nuclear antigens, purpura, polyarthritis, and so on. The disease usually affects young female dogs and often terminates in renal failure. No particular breed seems to have a predilection for developing canine SLE; all could develop the disease. The doctors have treated German shepherds, French poodles, Laborador retrievers, mongrel puppies, and others.

Dr. Schwartz explained that the dogs provide a unique opportunity to study the etiology (cause) and pathogenesis (origin) of systemic lupus erythematosus in a large nonhuman species. Blood samples from the dogs are taken at monthly intervals. The serum is analyzed for antibodies to nuclear antigens, using the LE cell tests, the fluorescent ANA test, and a radioactive assay for native and denatured DNA.

My original interview with Dr. Schwartz took place several years ago. Recently, I called Dr. Schwartz to ask him if he had found any new developments. He suggested that I talk with Dr. Fred Quimby, who was helping him with the research on lupus in dogs.

Like Dr. Lewis, Dr. Quimby is a veterinarian and an immunologist. He is currently director of Laboratory Animal Resources at Cornell University in New York. When he first started his work on canine lupus, in 1974, he had been associated with Dr. Lewis for one year.

"As you recall," Dr. Quimby said, "the dog colony was originally developed to study, among other things, whether systemic lupus can be inherited. Our most recent findings indicate that the disease could be genetically transmissible. But we know, from looking at the way these animals develop the disease, that the mechanism of inheritance is extremely complex and still unpredictable." He explained that the incidence of clinical SLE was greater in canine offspring with positive ANA and LE-cell tests, regardless of the clinical status of their parents. The offspring of two parents with clinical SLE have a higher incidence of SLE than the offspring of normal dogs; however, not all the offspring of SLE parents develop SLE. In addition, there have been offspring of two canine parents (which only had serologic evidence of lupus, i.e., ANA, LE cell, etc., but no clinical signs of disease) that did develop clinical SLE. This implies that each parent may contribute genetic factors which, by themselves, are not enough to cause clinical SLE, but which, together in the same dog, allow SLE to be expressed. The same results were demonstrated also in New Zealand black mice.

Another interesting phenomenon is that other non-SLE autoimmune diseases frequently develop in the offspring of parent dogs with SLE. This implies that the tendency to develop any autoimmune disease is inherited by a mechanism separate from that which dictates the precise disease. Dr. Quimby believes that multiple genes must be involved in the production of SLE in both dogs and humans.

Scientists have also observed that most dogs who have developed autoimmune disease have a defect in lymphocyte function. In these animals, the production of antibody is abnormally high. Dr. Quimby notes that this is also seen in both humans and mice with lupus.

Dr. Quimby's laboratory is also pursuing the latest virus theory. His interest in the subject was stimulated by a test conducted in his own lab. In this test the research team examined lymphocytes from both humans and dogs with SLE. To their amazement, the lymphocytes taken from patients with lupus had on their surface a substance similar to that found in certain viruses. Lymphocytes from normal people and dogs did not contain such a substance. In addition, tissues collected from cadavers of dogs with either SLE or another non-autoimmune disease were examined, using an entirely different method, and were found to contain large amounts of viral protein.

The presence of viral proteins does not necessarily indicate that a virus caused the lupus. One way to clarify this issue would be to recover a virus from dogs with lupus, and show that this virus will cause lupus in a normal dog.

Dr. Quimby said: "We have documentation that, in certain instances, microbes found in the environment may infect an individual, and that individual will subsequently develop an autoimmune disease. A strep throat may lead to rheumatic heart disease. This occurs when the patient makes antibodies against *Streptococcus*. These antibodies fail to recognize the difference between *Streptococcus* and heart muscle. So, in that particular instance, the patient's body is making an immune attack against an infectious agent and, at the same time, making an attack against his or her own body. A certain number of people who contract the virus responsible for infectious mononucleosis apparently also develop positive ANA. In dogs, and in some humans, bacterial infections may lead to the formation of circulating immune complexes that are subsequently deposited in the kidneys. This renal lesion would mimic lupus nephritis.

"The latent virus theory, however, is completely different. In this theory, the infectious agent may well be part of the individual's body from birth. The virus is not found in the environment, but, rather, is transferred from the parents to their offspring through genetic mechanisms."

Dr. Quimby showed me a few slides of lupus dogs. One slide was of a Shetland sheepdog called Lady. Lady had various systemic manifestations including central nervous system (CNS) involvement with personality changes. Three months before Dr. Quimby saw this dog, she was extremely friendly, and would often jump and cuddle up in a stranger's lap. Then, over a period of several months, Lady became extremely shy and would often run to a corner and shake when anyone approached her. The dog became withdrawn and began experiencing mild seizures. She also developed a temporary hearing and visual impairment.

Until recently, no confirmed cases were known of canine lupus with CNS involvement, but scientists now know that it exists. Even more recently, they have seen dogs with the classic butterfly rash. These dogs develop the rash if they are exposed to the sun. Researchers have observed this in Shetland sheepdogs with clinical and serological evidence of systemic lupus erythematosus. "Once you let these dogs roam in the sunshine, they develop a rash and also hair loss," Dr. Quimby said. He observed that the dog's rashes get better if they are kept indoors.

Another slide was of a Shetland sheepdog with discoid lupus. The dog had a lesion under its right eye. Dr. Quimby commented that the Shetland sheepdog appears to be a breed at risk for both SLE and discoid lupus. Also, some Shetlands with discoid lupus have subsequently developed systemic disease.

Interestingly, studies of dogs admitted to Angell Memorial Animal Hospital with SLE indicate that 90 percent of the female cases occurred in nonspayed females, although the total clinical population of female dogs includes 50 percent spayed dogs. Dr. Quimby said this may indicate that ovarectomy (removal of the ovaries) has a protective effect on the development of the disease in dogs. Literature indicating a similar effect in humans is scant.

Dr. Quimby has come across several dogs in which the major symptom of lupus was fatigue. Further observation of these animals uncovered a wide range of other symptoms, including simple muscular weakness and profound depression. Dr. Quimby and his colleagues identified at least three factors that may contribute to fatigue in dogs with SLE.

One, which has also been described in humans, is anemia. Many dogs with SLE are diagnosed initially with hemolytic anemia. The deficiency of circulating red cells leads to poor oxygenation of skeletal muscle, resulting in fatigue.

Another symptom of lupus in dogs is malnutrition. Dr. Quimby has seen several SLE dogs who have stopped eating. This led to malnutrition and, thus, to fatigue. Dr. Quimby explained that some dogs may stop eating because they develop ulcers in their mouths and along their intestinal tracts. Some dogs have had ulcerative colitis; rectal bleeding is common in these animals. In other instances, dogs have stopped eating with no evidence of ulceration. Some of these animals undergo a behavioral change that influences their eating habits. Some of the dogs studied by Dr. Quimby that had stopped eating began eating again if their standard diet was modified. Dr. Quimby explained that sometimes these dogs need a little coaching and tempting to get started again.

Along these same lines, Dr. Quimby has observed dogs with a loss of appetite because the lack of normal secretions from their salivary glands has led to a dry mouth and extensive dental cavities. The incidence of cavities in dogs is normally extremely low, unless some condition like this occurs. These dogs, with lupus and a reduction in salivary flow, might have a problem called Sjögren's syndrome.

A third factor that contributes to fatigue in a few dogs with SLE is polymyositis, inflammation of skeletal muscle. In dogs with this disease any movement elicits pain. One lupus dog has developed thyroiditis. This animal had an immune-mediated inflammation of the thyroid gland. In addition, Dr. Quimby said, the lack of thyroxine produced severe depression in the dog: "Speaking of fatigue, this dog was like a rug on the floor; he could not move." Once Dr. Quimby diagnosed the problem, he gave the dog Synthroid (a synthetic thyroxine), and the dog became active again.

Dr. Quimby postulated that the most important factor contributing to fatigue in dogs is inflammation of the joints. Similar to rheumatoid arthritis, this is the most common site of inflammation in dogs with SLE; 50 percent of lupus dogs have it. The inflammation in a dog's joint capsule strongly resembles the inflammation in both the thyroid gland and the muscle. According to Dr. Quimby, the inflammatory processes affecting different organs in the human lupus patient may look very similar.

Approximately 5 percent of dogs with SLE have thrombocytopenia (a deficiency of platelets). Dr. Quimby explained that these dogs bruise easily. During one examination, Dr. Quimby palpated the dog's abdomen to see if he could detect an enlarged spleen. Where he pressed the belly, the animal developed bruises. "This has taught us to be more gentle when we examine dogs with SLE," Dr. Quimby said.

Lupus seems to affect dogs' fertility. Dr. Quimby said, "In our dog colony we have observed two phenomena that may account for low birth rates. First, lupus dogs that have not been inbred display a certain incidence of spontaneous abortion and stillborn deliveries. I have noticed from breeding records of our Shetland sheepdogs that the average litter size appears abnormally low in families that have SLE. In our inbred colony we have observed major problems in reproduction. Many females remain unresponsive for years. When we studied this problem, we realized that many of these dogs had abnormalities in estrogen and progesterone production. We believe that the abnormal levels of estrogen and progesterone in the blood of these dogs may be associated with abnormal estrus cycles. Furthermore, abnormalities in the levels of these hormones in the pregnant female dog may interfere with proper implantation and fetal development, resulting in abortion."

Dr. Schwartz was very interested in the possibility that certain virus infections could be instrumental in the development of SLE. He had some support for this contention from an experiment conducted earlier with dogs. Dr. Schwartz's research team bred the same female and male dog three times and noticed that all the offspring developed autoantibodies by six months of age. Following the fourth breeding, the investigators delivered the puppies into a sterile isolator and found that at no time during the dogs' four-year residence did they develop autoantibodies. One of these puppies was removed and sent back to the dog colony to live with its mother and father. This dog developed antinuclear antibodies, LE cells, and autoimmune thyrogastric syndrome after six months. This is a single experiment that must be verified, but it does suggest that an environmental factor triggered the autoimmune disease.

Dr. Schwartz has also discovered that all dogs that develop clinical SLE have autoantibodies against their lymphocytes. Under the proper conditions, these antilymphocyte antibodies may cause profound decreases in a dog's circulating lymphocyte count. Dr. Schwartz's lab is currently investigating whether this autoantibody affects the canine immune system. Their current investigations involve measuring each of the different types of canine lymphocytes needed to produce an immune response, using monoclonal antibodies. Previous results in humans and mice have shown changes in certain populations of lymphocytes in patients with SLE. Dr. Schwartz would like to know if similar changes occur in dogs, and if these changes can be induced by antilymphocyte antibodies, infectious agents, drugs, and diet, or whether they must be inherited. Two new areas Dr. Schwartz's lab has been pursuing include autoimmune disease induced in cats with 6-propylthiouracil (6-PTU), and the influence of diet on survival and autoimmunity in mice.

Some time ago, Dr. Mark Peterson of the Animal Medical Center in New York City observed that some cats treated with 6-PTU for overactive thyroid glands developed anemia. Later he was able to show that these cats had autoantibodies to their red blood cells (Coombs antibody). Dr. Schwartz's lab was interested in how this drug, which is known to cause autoimmune disease in some otherwise normal humans, caused autoimmune disease in cats. Studies in normal cats showed that approximately 50 percent of all cats given the drug develop both Coombs antibody and antinuclear antibody. All cats develop autoimmune hemolytic anemia, and some develop autoimmune disease involving the liver and kidney. If the drug is discontinued, the cats get well. Most recently Dr. Schwartz discovered that when cats with 6-PTU-induced disease were given 6-propyluracil (6-PU) instead of 6-PTU, they all got better. This suggests that a very small area of the 6-PTU molecule, a single sulfur atom, is required for the maintenance of this autoimmune disease, since only this sulfur atom is missing in 6-PU.

Interest in the relationship between nutrition and immunity has been intense for some time; most recently, investigators have demonstrated increased life span in autoimmune-prone NZB and NZB/NZW mice on rations with reduced caloric intake. High-fat diets have also been shown to increase the severity of glomerulonephritis (a kidney disorder) and arteriosclerosis in these same mouse strains. Dr. David Mark and Dr. Marc Weksler at Cornell University Medical College have been studying the effect of restriction of high fat in diets fed to the MRL-1 strain of mouse. This strain also develops SLE with massive lymph-node enlargement by six months of age. It has been shown that calorie restriction increases survival, decreases the severity of kidney disease, and appears to decrease the level of circulating immune complexes in MRL-1 mice. However, in contrast to studies in NZB/NZW mice, researchers have been unable to show an increased incidence of vascular inflammation. When these mice were fed high-fat diets, they developed lipid-containing vascular lesions, similar to those associated with arteriosclerosis. The interrelationship between autoimmune disease, diet, and arterio-sclerosis is currently under investigation at Cornell University.

* * *

[4] The medical research community in Boston and the surrounding area includes many individuals who are working diligently to solve the mysteries of lupus. One is Dr. Dwight R. Robinson of Massachusetts General Hospital in Boston. A well-known clinician, Dr. Robinson is an associate professor of medicine at Harvard University Medical School and a physician at Massachusetts General Hospital. His interest in medical research concerns the mechanisms of inflammatory processes in rheumatic diseases.*

In a recent interview for *Lupus News*, Dr. Robinson stressed that kidney disease remains one of the major complications of systemic lupus. Although medication with prednisone and other immunosuppressant drugs is the generally accepted approach to treating lupus, in some patients the disease progresses in spite of these agents. Some new forms of treatment have been proposed, but they remain unproven. Dr. Robinson discussed plasmapheresis, which is currently undergoing experimental trials in SLE. "The purpose of this procedure is to remove autoantibodies and possibly other deleterious factors from the patient's circulation," Dr. Robinson said, and emphasized that at this time plasmapheresis is still experimental. Some individuals may have been benefited and the procedure holds some promise, but it cannot be recommended for general use since its safety and efficacy have not yet been established. Therefore, there remains a desperate need for the development of newer, more effective, and better tolerated forms of therapy in SLE, especially with regard to kidney involvement.

* * *

[5] According to Dr. Dwight Robinson of Massachusetts General Hospital, recent research has raised the possibility that a nutritional approach to the control of the inflammation in lupus may be possible under certain circumstances: "Physicians speak of the confusion as to the role of food in a variety of diseases and stress the need for

* Support from the Lupus Foundation of America, Inc., Massachusetts Chapter, has enabled Dr. Robinson to continue his experiments, which may lead to an improvement in lupus therapy.

solid scientific studies to provide reliable information to both the medical community and the general community. Off and on, one hears of claims for various diets in the treatment of arthritis and other diseases. Yet many of these remedies are unproven. At the present time there is no evidence that any dietary alteration affects the course or relieves the symptoms of any form of arthritis. However, there is a specific rationale for thinking that alterations in the fat or lipids in the diet might alter inflammatory reactions by modifying the synthesis of prostaglandins and related compounds, which may in turn affect lupus:

"A few years ago it was discovered that a group of Eskimos in northern Greenland, subsisting on fish and other seafood, had an alteration in the function of their blood platelets (the substances largely responsible for clotting) that was related to the fatty-acid composition of their diet. When these Eskimos were fed a diet containing plant lipid, the composition of fatty acids in their tissues was altered, which in turn altered the synthesis of prostaglandins by their blood platelets. This led to a mild bleeding defect of no serious clinical consequences, but pointed the way to observations indicating that prostaglandin metabolism was affected by dietary means. We reasoned, therefore, that if altering diet affected the synthesis of prostaglandins by platelets, it might affect the functions of prostaglandins in other areas."

Dr. Robinson's research team extrapolated from the experience with Greenland Eskimos and reasoned that if alteration of the dietary fatty acid can affect prostaglandins and their role in platelet function, it may be possible to modify prostaglandin function in other tissues in ways that may modify inflammatory reactions, such as those that occur with lupus. Therefore, his team embarked on a series of experiments with inflammatory models in experimental animals to determine whether by altering the animals' tissue lipid they could, through changes in metabolism of prostaglandins and related compounds, alter their inflammatory responses. One of these models was the NZB/NZW hybrid mouse, a well-accepted model for human systemic lupus. Dr. Robinson's initial experiments with these animals have demonstrated that a diet containing a high content of fish oil as a lipid source produces a dramatic prolongation of survival and protection from the renal disease that invariably develops in these animals.

Although Dr. Robinson stresses that it is a big extrapolation under any circumstances to draw conclusions about human diseases based on an animal model, he is optimistic because of the similarity of the mouse disease to human lupus. Serologic changes as well as histopathologic changes in the mice mimic human systemic lupus almost identically, and, in fact, many of the existing modes of treatment such as corticosteroids and cytotoxic drugs were developed based on experiments with this mouse model.

In another experiment, Dr. Robinson's lab delayed the introduction of the fish-oil-containing diet until the mice had developed overt renal disease, in order to develop a more accurate model for human lupus in the mice. Even under these circumstances the progression of the renal disease was definitely delayed in animals treated with fish oil compared to controlled diets.

Of course, swallowing fish oil does not seem like a very appetizing prospect. Said Dr. Robinson, "We clearly are not coming up with something that will make the pages of *Gourmet* magazine. However, based on our work with the lupus mice, we estimate that as little as one ounce of fish oil per day taken in divided doses might provide substantial benefit to patients with systemic lupus and kidney involvement. At this point no diets have been developed for human consumption, but purification of the fish oil removes much of the undesirable smell and taste. Furthermore, since a diet high in fish oil has been taken regularly for centuries by Eskimos without apparent deleterious effects, we presume it will be safe for human consumption. In addition, the oil administered would contain only three or four hundred calories per day and allow patients to ingest an otherwise completely normal diet. Finally, it would be desirable to isolate the specific protective factor in the fish oil that confers the beneficial effect, and further work in our laboratories is needed to pursue this question. Only a very small amount of a purified natural compound isolated from the fish oil might be the appropriate treatment."

In conclusion, Dr. Robinson pointed out that researchers have an example of a possible new approach to the control of the inflammatory reaction that leads to kidney damage in human systemic lupus. "So far," he cautioned, "the results are based entirely on an experimental animal model, and it cannot be concluded that this approach will be successful in the treatment of the human disease." According to Dr. Robinson, plans are being made for a clinical trial involving several academic centers, to begin in the near future, and it is hoped that some definitive information about the possible benefits of this approach to the treatment of human lupus will be available soon thereafter.

Dr. Robinson's latest research has concentrated on four areas of the fish-oil problem.

In the first set of experiments, Dr. Robinson's lab obtained a highly purified eicosapentaenoic acid (EPA) ethyl ester, which is being administered to groups of NZB/NZW mice to determine the effects of a purified fatty acid on the course of their lupuslike kidney disease. The rationale for this study is that EPA is one of the unusual fatty acids in fish oil that was previously demonstrated to protect mice from lupuslike kidney disease. It is necessary to determine the protective factor of fish oil in order to make possible clinical applications of these findings more feasible, as well as to provide a basis for understanding the mechanisms of the protective effects of fish oil. This research is still underway.

Dr. Robinson's efforts to purify fatty acids from fish oil have been unsuccessful to date, and his researchers have abandoned this aspect of the project as not feasible. Fortunately, they have been successful in obtaining purified fatty acids from other sources, and these will be tested for their ability to protect against kidney disease.

Dr. Robinson's lab has also tested reversal of established kidney disease in NZB/NZW mice. This experiment has successfully demonstrated that institution of the fish-oil diets, even after proteinuria (protein in the urine) and kidney disease had developed in the NZB/NZW mice, still resulted in a prolongation of the life span of these animals and, in some cases, apparent reversal of the progression of the disease. This conclusion is based on examination of kidney tissue as well as observation of the mice's life span and measurements of protein excretion in their urine. This study leads to the conclusion that the fish-oil diet is therapeutic as well as prophylactic for kidney disease and suggests that clinical application of this approach to the treatment of lupus nephritis is feasible.

In a fourth set of studies, Dr. Robinson's lab carried out successful experiments demonstrating that addition of graded doses of fish oil to diets protects against kidney disease. The initial fish-oil content of the mice's diet was 49 percent of the total caloric intake, which demonstrated clearly protective effects. Similar protective effects were observed when the total oil content was reduced to 25 percent of the total caloric value of the diet, and partial protection was observed when the fish-oil content was reduced to 10 percent of the caloric content of the diet. Thus, Dr. Robinson has determined a dose-response relationship of the diet to protection from kidney disease that indicates a diminution of the protective effect at a content of 10 percent of the total caloric intake. These findings will be considered as guidelines for future clinical trials.

Dr. Robinson hopes that in a year or two he may have some conclusive findings that will determine whether this is a promising approach in treating humans.

4

Why Lupus Is More Common in Women Than in Men

I wrote my first book on lupus, *The Sun Is My Enemy*, in 1972, after reading in a national magazine the word *Help* in large letters over the picture of a woman whose face was covered with gauze. The caption read: "I suffer from an obscure human ailment called systemic lupus erythematosus." I recall reading those words over and over and feeling a deep compassion for that woman. I understood only too well her helplessness and desperation, and I tried to find her. Days later I went back to look for the ad, but the magazine was gone. I dedicated *The Sun Is My Enemy* to this woman, and to all the other women who are struck by lupus. I thought then, as I still do, that women have been stigmatized for much too long by an illness with an unpronounceable name, an unknown cause, and an unclear prognosis.

For centuries women with lupus have been the unwitting victims of their own environment—of the sun and of drugs—and they have had to cope with unusual burdens. In the words of Dr. Patricia Fraser of Harvard University Medical School and Brigham and Women's Hospital in Boston:

> When voluntary consciousness-raising is fashionable, women with lupus may not have this option. The demands of this disease on a woman's life often prevent a leisurely

61

consideration of her appropriate role or roles in life and force rapid, painful confrontation with the conflicting signals society sends to women.

One of the most treacherous and yet most effective tools of women's socialization is the media. The ideal woman portrayed by the media is a superficial plastic doll with long, flowing or "short and sassy," but nevertheless thick, shining hair, with flawless skin and very subtle curves to her body. As part of her normal development and evolution of self, each woman learns to recognize this myth for what it is and to take pride in her particular body and soul composition, no matter how unlike the media's standard. This gradual transition may be interrupted when lupus strikes in adolescence, as it often does, or in early adulthood. The woman may not yet come to like herself as she is. Superimposed on this arrested development may be bodily malfunctions that, according to media indoctrination, are severe impediments to the ideal—especially skin rash and hair loss. Perhaps the most serious threat to body image as we are told to see it is cortisone therapy. How many women have rejected this therapy or have regulated their doses unbeknownst to their doctors in a desperate attempt to avoid the well-known side effects? A woman with lupus may well understand the need for this medication; nevertheless, the external forces of society may force her to undermine her own self-interest of better health.

The cause of feminism also takes its toll on lupus patients. It urges the woman of the 1980s to be all things—wife, mother, athlete, executive. It fosters the image of the tireless, crusading superwoman who is capable of anything she sets her mind to. For most of us non-superwomen in good health, the discrepancy between the real and the ideal is clear and the ideal is used as a guideline to modify our lives. During periods of high energy and heightened motivation we may attempt to emulate features of the superwoman, but as we fatigue we drop back to somewhere near or slightly above where we started. Nothing is lost and something is gained in the experience; no harm is done.

With lupus the issues and stakes are always higher, the risks magnified. I recall a woman in her forties who had stable lupus for many years. Each summer she would visit relatives on Cape Cod and spend a leisurely summer. One sunny June, in 1978, she felt her husband should no longer be responsible for her financial needs in their vacation period and that she should support herself. As an unskilled laborer she set out doing odd jobs, spending long hours in the sun mowing lawns, tidying yards, and the like. Much to her surprise and dismay she made little money and developed a lupus flare related to the sudden exposure. Perhaps this is an extreme example, but it illustrates a common dilemma. For the woman without lupus the burst of new independence would either be enjoyed or used to put the marriage relationship in perspective, or both. For this woman with lupus it accomplished only one thing—more lupus.

Do not mistake my tone. A woman with lupus is not the most unfortunate person in the world. She is not the total victim. The additional stress this illness places on the woman frequently builds self-image, restores perspective on society. Women with lupus often become strong women out of necessity.

The use of the word *lupus* to describe the chronic inflammatory disease that preferentially affects women illustrates the subconscious apprehension felt by generations of physicians who have managed these patients. The trepidation fostered by lupus is illustrated in the very term used to describe the condition. Some of the first observers compared the facial lesions to the bite of a wolf, while others likened the rash to the facial mask of a wolf.

The patients who live with this malady are no less fearful. The weight of unanswered questions presses heavily on them. "What causes lupus?" This is usually the first of many frustrating questions without an answer. Patients who are told, "You have a mild form of lupus," correctly inquire, "Will it get worse?" As the patient endures a prolonged flare she (or he) may ask, "When will I ever get better?" An uneasiness also punctuates the existence of the lupus patient who has been free of symptoms for months or years and gives rise to the inquiry, "How long will this remission last?"

I have heard patients say, "I'd rather die than go on looking like this." It is difficult, especially for the young, not to be brainwashed into believing that they must always be beautiful, or energetic, or independent, and never look like they might need help. Eventually, however, we learn that every person needs help at one time or another, that we need to save energy for self-development and adjustment.

I have received scores of letters from patients describing their uncertainties and asking questions about their fears and tribulations so they can find the strength to survive.

Diana is a young patient from Wisconsin with whom I have corresponded. She tells a moving story of a life that is exasperating and full of uncertainties. Diana writes:

Often I feel alone with this disease. My friends and family tell me to quit worrying about it, and my husband, who is unfortunately no support at all, thinks I'm a hypochondriac. It's all quite overwhelming at times, and your letter really brightened my day.

I am afraid of the future. I try so hard to have positive thoughts and I've gotten to be an expert at showing my strongest side, but most of the time I'm terrified! I don't want my fears to consume me, and I realize that I could easily become an emotional cripple. I truly do believe that faith and positive thinking can make all the difference in the world and I try to live each day accordingly, but then I have a day where I feel absolutely lousy and the fear returns; I realize that I have lupus. I analyze myself constantly and have realized that my worst fear is of the disease being progressive.

I have read in several articles that lupus is a progressive disease, and yet my doctors tell me that this is not necessarily true. I worry then that they're padding the truth so I'll feel better. Mrs. Aladjem, someone told me that very often the disease remains the same as it is within the first couple of years. If that is true then I'll relax, knowing that thus far only my skin seems to be affected. Reading about its progressiveness throws me off again, though.

I am at the point now where every symptom I ever feel worries me. Last week, for example, I felt like a dishrag. My eyes were puffy, I had no energy, I wanted to stay in bed and pull the blankets up over my head to sleep until I felt like Diana again. Maybe it was from the lupus and maybe it wasn't. It worried me to death, though, because right away the word "progressive" jumped at me.

I need a job desperately, but part of me is afraid to get

one. I'm always reading about how important it is to get enough rest. I'm afraid that if I get a full-time job my lupus will get worse.

I'm treating myself like a sick person even when I feel fine, and I don't want to be doing this, but I'm so scared and unsure about what to expect.

This summer is better than last summer, but I still have such a long way to go. Last July when lupus was diagnosed I cried each morning as the sun streamed through my window. I'd always worshipped the sun, and all of a sudden it was like an evil monster. This year I'm back to loving the sun, but at a safe distance. I'm hoping that with every day it'll get easier. I want to believe that I can live a long happy life and be basically healthy, and yet I don't believe in false hope.

Are my doctors telling me the truth when they say I'll probably never be any worse off than I am right now? Or are they just trying to make my load lighter? Are they correct in saying I'll probably not die from lupus? Or are they trying to instill wishful thinking into my head? My internist calls it cutaneous, my dermatologist refers to it as discoid, and yet I feel at times like a truck ran over me. ("Totally drained" about sums it up.) I am a worrier when it comes to my health, which makes me wonder if I'm not perhaps bringing on some of my own symptoms. It's a merry-go-round, as you can see, and I don't mean to ramble on, but I want to have you understand what I'm saying.

If you can shed any light on these ever-present fears of mine, I'd welcome your comments. I don't want to pester you, but I want so desperately to reach some peace of mind and go on with my life instead of dwelling on my health.

P.S.: For awhile I worried that my kidneys were involved and I'd die. I don't fear that anymore because I read that if the kidneys aren't affected within the first two years then they won't be. All tests show that my kidneys are fine.

Now I worry constantly that I have brain involvement! My hands and feet tingle and fall asleep a lot, which terrifies me, and I have anxiety (or panic) attacks, which I worry may be due to CNS involvement. Good grief, will I become psychotic? Yes, I do, indeed, worry a lot.

I read and listen to the patients' stories and I grieve over them. Listening may be the only contribution I have been able to make to patients. Some think it helps. However, over the years I have grown to recognize the pain that lingers in the women's eyes. I can recognize the characteristic expressions that come from years of suffering. The expressions change from anger to envy or jealousy, to resentment, to melancholy, and, finally, to resignation. The look in the patients' eyes possesses a secret of the illness that doctors are ignoring. Through letters like Diana's, we are making this understanding available to them. But are they willing to listen? Are they ready to hear the truth they have not yet accepted? Should doctors listen to patients even when the physicians' convictions and laboratory testing lead them to different conclusions? Should the patients' grievances be explored in depth, considered for the sake of those who are ill and need counsel and treatment? The uniqueness of lupus is ours—and ours alone; and at the core remains the question about why so many women are suffering from this disease.

I asked Dr. Norman Talal, professor of medicine and microbiology and head of the division of clinical immunology at the University of Texas Health Center in San Antonio, why lupus is more prevalent in women. I also asked him to explain the relationship between immunology and autoimmune diseases such as lupus. Dr. Talal answered that autoimmune diseases may arise as an abnormality in a system based on self-recognition. These diseases can be linked to many factors. Not all of the factors are known yet, nor do we understand how they interact, nor which ones are most important. According to Dr. Talal, immune regulation depends on the proper functioning of immune response genes and on maintaining a balance between subsets of T and B lymphocytes. In systemic lupus erythematosus (SLE), T-cell function tends to be decreased and B-cell activity tends to be excessive. He pointed out that clinical medicine provides numerous examples of autoantibody production without autoimmune disease. Certain drugs, some infectious diseases, and the process of aging itself may be associated with a limited form of autoimmunity; upon successful eradication of the infection, or discontinuation of the offending drug, the symptoms of the autoimmune disease disappear.

Dr. Talal also explained the meaning of immunoendocrinology, and discussed the relationship between immunology and endocrinology, and the ability of sex hormones to modulate the autoimmune disorder. Immunoendocrinology refers to the science of studying the interactions between these two important systems. Dr. Talal first became interested in this area of research when he and his colleagues worked on studies showing that male and female hormones influence the lupuslike disease that affects a strain of mice called NZB/NZW. Androgens, male hormones, and estrogens, female hormones, are small molecules that enter cells and influence their behavior. A simple male hormone is necessary for developing male characteristics. Many studies of sex hormones have shown greater immune responses in females than in males.

This may have a bearing on why lupus is more common in women than in men, a phenomenon that was noticed from the earliest days when lupus was first being diagnosed. Moreover, the difference seems to depend on the presence or absence of the menstrual cycle. For example, if one considers only young children prior to the onset of menses, or postmenopausal women, the ratio of female to male patients with lupus is approximately 2½ to 1. However, women in their childbearing years are ten times more likely to develop SLE than men.

The classical animal model for studying lupus is the New Zealand black and white F_1 (NZB/NZW) mouse. This strain of mice was first introduced into experimental medicine in the 1950s and has been an important mainstay of research on lupus ever since. As in human patients, the disease in NZB/NZW mice also shows a marked female predominance. For example, female NZB/NZW mice develop the clinical and laboratory features of lupus several months earlier than males. This gives the medical investigator an opportunity to study the influence of sex hormones on lupus.

Dr. Talal and his associates have been investigating the role of hormones in lupus for the past several years. Their first experiments were designed to see whether the presence of the testes, which secrete androgens, might protect male mice from lupus. This might explain the delay before contracting the disease shown in male NZB/NZW mice. In order to study this question, they performed prepubertal sterilization on both male and female mice. The castrated males developed an accelerated form of lupus that was indistinguishable from the disease form in their female counterparts. By contrast, the removal of the ovaries did not significantly influence the course of disease in the female mice.

Next, male hormones were injected into female mice, and for

the first time a significant therapeutic influence was detected. The female mice receiving androgen developed very few features of lupus, whereas mice of both sexes given estrogen developed the disease quickly. These results seemed to confirm the suspicion that androgens were protective, and that estrogens accelerate the development of lupus in mice.

To explore the applicability of these results in a clinical situation, Dr. Talal and his associates performed a series of experiments in which androgen treatment was delayed until an age when the mice had already contracted the lupuslike disease. Dr. Talal says that even under these circumstances, in which the progress of the disease would make treatment difficult, the therapeutic effect of male hormone was again observed. Thus, the sum of their experimental findings strongly points to the conclusion that androgen has a protective influence.

Dr. Talal is exploring the influence of androgen on specific lymphocyte functions and subpopulations of lymphocytes, the effect on macrophages, and the effect on immune complexes and on how they are eliminated from the immune system. The most interesting results to date suggest that androgens promote the removal of immune complexes from the blood, and may prevent their deposition in the kidneys. Such a mechanism would result in less glomerulonephritis, a form of kidney inflammation, and might prevent the development of uremia, a kidney disorder in which urea and other substances are retained in the blood.

According to Dr. Talal, androgen therapy has not yet been tried in patients with lupus, because of the masculinizing side effects of such treatment. However, he and his associates have investigated the possibility that a nonmasculizing androgen might have therapeutic effects in NZB/NZW mice. Unfortunately, this preparation has not proven effective, and therefore they could not endorse its use in patients.

However, despite the apparent role of sex hormones, patients with lupus seem no more likely to be sterile or impotent than the average person.

Dr. Talal emphasizes that we are living in a time of great discovery (especially in the field of immunology), and he stresses the rapidity with which creative thinking is translated into scientific observations in immunology, which has made it difficult even for workers in the field to keep abreast of the latest developments. Is there any newer information available regarding why lupus is more common in women? Dr. Talal wrote me an engaging letter on this question.

I am hastening to respond to your request for more information regarding why lupus is more common in women. I wonder if you would not like to use for your chapter the following quotation from Sonnet 24 of William Shakespeare:

"Thou art thy mother's glass, and she in thee
Calls back the lovely April of her prime."

I think it is so beautiful and expressive of both femininity and the unfortunate price women pay with an increased incidence of autoimmune disease.

Last summer in Kyoto, Japan, at the International Immunology Congress, I presented a paper representing the extension of our work on sex steroid hormones. Basically, many diseases have now been shown to be suppressed by androgen or accelerated by estrogen. These include thyroiditis, myasthenia gravis, and arthritis, in addition to lupus. We have very good evidence that female hormones weaken suppressor mechanisms while male hormones maintain them. This is probably one of the major mechanisms whereby "femaleness" tends to predispose toward autoimmunity. I believe that the immunologic hyperresponsiveness of normal females may be related to reproductive immunology insofar as it may allow the female to manifest immunologic mechanisms that protect the fetus from rejection. . . .

The brain and the immune system are two nonclassic target organs for sex hormone action. In the brain, sex hormones influence such things as sexual attractiveness (e.g., bird songs), reproductive behavior, aggression, and territorial defense. Thus, all of these favor survival of the species. I want to argue by analogy that sex hormone effects on reproductive immunology also favor species survival by allowing what is essentially a foreign graft (the fetus) to be carried to term and delivered as a healthy baby.

This kind of thinking also represents an extension of the concept of immunoendocrinology discussed before. I would now extend this to cover the interrelationships between three areas: the immune system, the classical endocrine system, and the neuroendocrine system, which is part of the brain. All three systems are mutually interactive and interdependent. Mood and emotions influence immunity in many ways, in part through the actions of specific neuropeptides, like endorphins, for which there are receptors on lymphocytes. I believe that, through sound immunologic mechanisms, depression or elation can affect immunoregulation and, therefore, autoimmune disorders. We certainly will be seeing increasing emphasis on this area in lupus research during the next decade.

Our own current interest in the interleukin-2 deficiency that develops in lupus patients can be considered another example of immunoendocrinology. Interleukin-2, or T-cell growth factor, is an immune hormone secreted by helper/inducer T cells that acts to influence many different circuits in the immune response. I hope we will find some of these immune factors or hormones to be therapeutic in lupus, and usher in a new era of immunotherapy that will avoid the dangerous and nonspecific complications of corticosteroids in immunosuppressive drugs. With God's will this will come true.

PART II

MANAGING LUPUS

5

The Doctor-Patient Partnership

Dr. T. Stephen Balch, director of the Jacqueline McClure Lupus Treatment Center in Atlanta, Georgia, has compiled some helpful tips about how to get the most from your doctor.

The relationship between you and your doctor is an integral aspect of your health care. It must continually improve so you benefit the most from it. It is not easy. Sometimes you may feel cooperation is difficult, that you are at odds with your doctor and have different interests. For example, you may want to hear more about your disease, while your doctor may have to hurry to another patient. Or you do not want to take a medication because of its side effects, while your doctor recommends it because he or she wants your disease to improve.

The key to a good doctor-patient relationship is realizing that you and your doctor are on the same team. The effort must go both ways. The physician needs to be confident that the patient is capable of becoming an actively participating partner in the decision-making process. You, the patient, will have to accept some of the responsibility for the results of medical decisions and see to it that you carry them out properly.

In former times, doctors gave people very little information about their illnesses and expected blind obedience to their instructions. Today we know that good compliance depends on a complete understanding of instructions and the patient's agreement that the final treatment plan is a good one and can be accepted by both members of the partnership.

The partnership improves as you realize that you are the one in charge of your body. You know how it feels, responds to different treatment, and changes with illness. You are also the one to see that you treat it right; only you can see that the treatment is carried out correctly. Try not to assume you cannot understand what is going on in your body.

Patients also need to realize that the doctor is just as subject to the same moods, pressures, and errors that they are. There is no reason to be intimidated by your doctor, or to follow orders blindly.

The following are some specific encounters you are likely to have with your doctor, with tips on how to make the best of them. These encounters include the initial office visit, the physical examination, your time between appointments, and a variety of other matters in the doctor-patient relationship.

THE INITIAL VISIT

In order to be the most productive at this visit, come prepared to explain your health state and why you are seeking medical help. Bring a legible list of your symptoms, the things that are bothering you, and of the points you want to discuss with your doctor. Be as concise and precise as possible. Hand the list to the doctor if you want. This way, he or she can go over everything much more quickly without either of you worrying that you will forget something important.

At this visit, tell your doctor about all the medications you are taking. You also need to mention any over-the-counter drugs you take; they could interfere with medication prescribed for you. If you keep a chart of your medication, bring it with you.

When seeing a patient for the first time, many physicians have no record of previous laboratory work or medical evaluations. They may waste a lot of time and money repeating tests that have been done before, perhaps recently. To avoid this situation, bring as many of your previous records of laboratory work or evaluations as you can. It is very important to remember that these test results may vary from time to time and from laboratory to laboratory. Attempts are currently being made to standardize many of the tests used with the lupus patient, and the laboratory your doctor uses should meet these standards. Also, bring a list of the names and addresses of your other doctors. And never assume that all the relevant information is in the records. Your memory and any record you may keep yourself are important sources of facts.

THE COMPREHENSIVE EXAMINATION OR "PHYSICAL"

You can help the doctor gain useful information during the physical examination by understanding that he or she is looking for specifics. Doctors are not mind readers. They learn much from you by blood tests, physical examinations, and other procedures, but a large part of the information they rely on to diagnose and treat must come from you. Doctors try to understand what is going on in you from your symptoms. Therefore, they need your input and observations. Be as specific as possible about how and what you are feeling and thinking.

After the physical, your physician should discuss your treatment options with you. For some people, the recommended treatment may be no more than adequate rest. For others, the treatment may involve medications, skin care, alteration of daily activities, physical or occupational therapy sessions, or home exercises. (Therapy sessions and home exercises will differ greatly from patient to patient, so the physician and patient must discuss them individually.) The exact combination will determine your treatment plan. To arrive at it, your doctor needs to understand such factors as eating and work habits, exercise preferences, outside interests, etc.

Your doctor should also tell you the best ways to take your medications—for example, if you should take them with meals, or what might happen if you change your dosage on your own. Your doctor should explain the side effects you may incur. Some are potentially dangerous; however, most are merely annoyances. Often physicians know ways to handle side effects that may occur.

Finally, it is often helpful to have your doctor explain to you how your medication works. For example, aspirin decreases pain and inflammation. The more informed you are about your care, the more successful your treatment will be.

BETWEEN OFFICE VISITS

You will help your doctor evaluate how well your treatment plan is working if you keep track of your progress and follow his or her instructions closely. Record your responses for discussion at your next visit. In particular, pay attention to what factors make you feel worse or better, and note when you take your medications and how they seem to affect you. Consider if your treatment plan may need to be changed. This may be necessary if you are having trouble following directions; you are having unpleasant side effects; you cannot afford the medication; or you are getting worse instead of better. Do not be afraid to ask your doctor to change your treatment; he or she will probably want to change something if you explain what is wrong.

If the medication becomes too expensive for you, look into ways to lower medication costs. One way is to ask your doctor about the possibility of prescribing generic or non-brand name drugs. These are often the same as brand-name drugs. You may also be able to get discounts on medications through an organization such as the American Association of Retired Persons. (They can be reached at 1909 K St., N.W., Washington, DC 20049; (202) 728-4300.)

OTHER ENCOUNTERS
AND ASPECTS OF THE PARTNERSHIP

Medical explanations are an area in which a perfect match between doctor and patient is difficult to achieve and describe. Each situation is unique. Different doctors handle medical discussions with their patients in different ways, and individual patients have different needs and expectations from their doctors.

Both the doctor and the patient should feel free to bring up the topic of referral for another opinion. Your partnership has little to lose and often much to gain by obtaining a second opinion, to keep your diagnosis and treatment based on the best possible information. After you have seen the second doctor, you should talk to your regular physician and discuss any changes in your treatment plan based on this consultation.

CONCLUSION

Physicians must set aside their image of themselves as the ones making crucial medical decisions alone, and instead undertake the less glamorous, more time-consuming process of exploring options and outcomes with the patient. Physicians often do not have specific training in participatory decision-making, and the methods of identifying a particular patient's preferences vary. Nonetheless, both the physician and the patient should make thoughtful efforts to spell out the values that affect their decisions. It is surprising to learn not only how revealing such dialogue is, but how effectively it creates a spirit of mutual trust. The team is complementary: you know a lot more about your body than the doctor does, and he or she knows more about medicine than you do. The key is to work *together* toward the goal of controlling a very difficult disease and improving your life as a result.

6

Lupus and Medications

Since early childhood, I have shown a sensitivity to medications. The drugs I took, instead of helping, caused problems, which were never interpreted correctly. The reactions should have been received as a warning signal from nature, not just for one drug, but for all the ineffective medication I received then. Now I am even afraid of aspirin. Yet for nearly twenty years I swallowed new pills and took injections passively, without thinking twice. I should have learned from experience, but I had to be hit over the head with the allergic reactions many, many times before reaching the right conclusions.

When I had active lupus, I was treated with large doses of cortisone, which led to retention of fluids. To alleviate the discomfort, I was given diuretics (water pills). The diuretics contained sulfonamides, which, I suspect, caused more harm than good. (Such diuretics continue to be prescribed by doctors who are unware of the potential harm caused by sulfonamides in lupus patients.) For the pains and aches I was taking aspirin, sometimes as many as sixteen per day. For the stomach distress, I took atropine, pyrabenzamine, Gelusil, and others. For my chronic sore throat, I was given small doses of penicillin and tetracycline.

Along with these drugs, the doctors instituted white cell injections (5 cc each time), niacin injections (1 cc per day), and autogenous vaccines (vaccines made from the patient's own bacteria). None of these are used any longer. I also took potassium chloride, vitamins B6 and B12, ascorbic acid (vitamin C), and folic acid. Today, doctors

78

are adding to the list of drugs, and tranquilizers are often recommended.

In 1953, medical specialists knew little about the toxicity or side effects of the steroids, the antimalarial drugs, or some of the other experimental medications that were given in the hope that they would alter the course of the disease. The lupus patient has to accept the immediate side effects of the drugs, as well as the side effects that may not occur until years after a specific drug has been taken.

In lupus, the list of experimental drugs is frighteningly large, and the question of what drugs are prescribed by the physician often depends on which research center you go to, and who the attending physician is.

I met with Dr. Stephen Kaplan, a professor of medicine at Brown University Medical School and chief of rheumatology at Roger Williams General Hospital in Providence, Rhode Island, and asked him to identify some of the drugs being used in the treatment of lupus today.

Dr. Kaplan said, "I think we ought to address several general issues before discussing some of the specific characteristics of the drugs that are used in the treatment of systemic lupus erythematosus (SLE). Remember, many of the manifestations of SLE are treatable. Some medications affect the mechanisms of the disease and alter the signs and symptoms of SLE. Many of these therapeutic agents actually treat the disease process and should not be considered just symptomatic treatment. In addition to the use of medications to treat the mechanisms of SLE, we are also able to treat some of the complications of SLE through advances in other areas of medical science, such as the recognition and treatment of infectious diseases and improved care in intensive or critical care units. The treatment of SLE is complicated by the wide variety of its signs and symptoms, as well as by the varying degrees of severity manifested in different individuals at any time. Unfortunately, among those patients whose involvement with SLE affects their kidneys or central nervous system, there are some whose disease will not be affected or controlled by currently available medical means. In dealing with these severe problems, we reach the frontiers of modern therapeutics and, when faced with such critical medical circumstances, we must carefully judge the point at which the chances of helping the individual with the aggressive use of potent medications become outweighed by the chances of doing harm. These considerations of 'doing no harm,' even in apparently extreme situations, have taken on added significance as we appreciate that improvement, such as in the supportive care of patients with central nervous system disease, may provide a critical period of time in which some spontaneous improvement may occur. In patients with the severest forms of renal disease in SLE, these considerations have assumed added importance with the development of a technology capable of providing kidney dialysis or even kidney transplantation."

Dr. Kaplan stresses that no cure for lupus is known at this time. However, he says, curability is not always a simple concept, and most serious illnesses, such as diabetes mellitus or common types of heart disease, may not be curable today but can frequently be controlled sufficiently to permit a normal life-style. Treatability, therefore, should be emphasized in disorders like SLE, so that patients and their physicians can work toward realistic expectations, and not be unnecessarily tormented or driven by overly optimistic or pessimistic notions. Dr. Kaplan believes that, whatever the treatment, it should include the intelligent use of preventative measures by the patient, such as appropriate screening from the sun when photosensitivity is a problem (see Chapter 7) and maintaining the warmth of the hands when Raynaud's phenomenon (spasm of the arteries of the fingers resulting in poor circulation) is present.

Medications and drugs, however, play a central role in dealing with the treatable manifestations of SLE. Without doubt, most medications that are used in lupus and other serious medical problems are double-edged swords. Their potential for producing significant beneficial effects must be considered in balance with their potential for producing adverse effects and added problems for the patient. We are all aware of the great feats a skilled mechanic can accomplish in repairing complex machinery with the proper tools, and, by contrast, we can also imagine the harm that can be done by the same tools, including the proverbial monkey wrench, when they have been applied improperly or carelessly. In medical therapeutics, medications act as highly developed specialized tools that have the capacity to alter complex reactions in a way that benefits the patient. Since these tools must function independently, the skill in their use comes in choosing the appropriate medication for the appropriate problem and prescribing the dosage that will produce a beneficial effect.

Because of the side effects of the various drugs given in the treatment of lupus, the patient may not always take the medications in the proper dosage. It is therefore critical for the patient to follow the physician's instructions about taking the medications as prescribed.

Dr. Kaplan said, "Patients need to maintain a level of the prescribed medications sufficient to affect the mechanisms of SLE. Since the body is continually inactivating and eliminating the drugs, maintaining a desirable effect by a drug depends on cooperation by the patient. Taking the medication so that the effect is fairly continuous prevents SLE from returning or gaining the upper hand. This must be balanced, of course, by the potential for each drug to produce adverse or side effects. One must keep the potential for these side effects in proper perspective. The principle in selecting the specific medication and the strength of the dosage for the appropriate medical problem should be in keeping with a sentiment expressed in Gilbert and Sullivan's *Mikado*: Let the [potential] punishment fit the crime. Clearly, all patients should be knowledgeable about the medications they are administering to themselves. If a side effect does appear, changing the dosage or shifting to an equivalent but different medication should follow deliberation involving both patient and physician."

Before discussing which medications are used in the treatment of lupus, it is important to understand that every medication has three names. Each drug has a precise chemical name that is usually very complicated and is generally not well known except to chemists working in the laboratory. Thus, each drug is also given a generic name, which is, in a sense, a shorthand for the complicated chemical name. The generic name refers to a specific medication, regardless of manufacturer. The third name for each drug is the trade name, which is the name a manufacturer uses to identify its particular product. In some states, laws mandate that if a drug is prescribed by its generic name, the least expensive generic equivalent carried by the pharmacy must be used to fill the prescription. All drugs in this chapter will be referred to by their generic names.

Corticosteroids

Many lupus patients take various forms of cortisone, and some experience adverse effects from long-term regular usage. There are now new drugs available to replace cortisone. According to Dr. Kaplan, after cortisone and its properties were discovered, many different forms of this drug were created in the laboratory, such as prednisone, prednisolone, triamcinolone, and others. These are generally stronger than the original chemical, but all have the same problems with respect to adverse effects. Physicians refer to all these forms of cortisone as steroids or corticosteroids, and corticosteroids are among the most potent drugs known to suppress inflammation. Steroids may also affect the cells of the immune system. In lupus, a disturbance in the regulation of the immune system eventually results in the inappropriate inflammatory activity responsible for many of the signs and symptoms of lupus. Because of this, the powerful antiinflammatory effect of steroids may be used in various manners in the management of lupus.

Steroid creams are successful in controlling skin rashes of lupus in addition to the ulcers that may appear in the nose, and such creams can often prevent the serious scarring that once characterized the progression of this manifestation of SLE. Prolonged use of some of the newer and more powerful forms may, over a period of time, do injury to the skin, however, so patients should discuss the situation with their physicians when prolonged usage of this topical medication is recommended. Some steroid preparations may be injected directly into a joint, says Dr. Kaplan, if the arthritis of SLE continues to be active in spite of other measures. Physicians worry about doing harm to a patient with steroid therapy not so much with its topical or intraarticular (within the joint) use as when the medication is administered on a regular basis over a long period of time.

I asked Dr. Kaplan to explain what cortisone compounds are.

"Cortisone compounds are hormones that are normally produced by the adrenal gland in each of us every day. Most of the time a fairly constant amount is produced each day, but when placed under stress, our bodies require increased amounts of these materials to maintain the metabolism that supports the blood pressure, maintains a normal balance of chemicals in the blood, and so on. A primary control for the amount of cortisone the adrenal glands produce is another hormone called adrenocorticotropic hormone (ACTH), which is produced by the pituitary gland at the base of the skull. One way to produce increased amounts of cortisone, therefore, is to administer increased amounts of ACTH by injection. This is a simple substitute for the administration of steroids, but it has little or no particular advantage over the more easily administered steroid pills. Cortisone is an important part of the metabolic systems in our body, and affects the stores of body sugar, protein, and fats, so as to help maintain an adequate supply and balance of these nutrients. Cortisone also affects the balance of chemicals in the blood that are important in maintaining normal blood pressure and hydration. Although many of these side effects are not dependent on exactly the same actions as the antiinflammatory effects of the steroids, the antiinflammatory activity has not yet been isolated from the activity on the metabolic systems. In particular, when an individual must take high doses of steroids in order to control the inflammation of a disease like SLE, the dosage produces an exaggerated effect on the various metabolic systems, with many consequences for the patient. Thus, steroid use should be thoroughly discussed by the patient and physician when these drugs are required to manage SLE."

Flannery O'Connor, the southern author who died from lupus in 1964, wrote that when she was on steroids, her face became round like a watermelon. There was a time when I looked like that myself (Figure 9). Dr. Kaplan explained that the impact of steroids on the metabolic system may include redistribution of the fatty stores of the body, causing the face to become round, the so-called moon face. The steroids can also raise the blood sugar above normal, increase appetite (which may result in weight gain), cause some weakening of the bony structures because of interference with calcium metabolism, increase the risk of developing infections, produce cataracts, etc. Many people, however, do take therapeutically beneficial amounts of steroids and experience relatively few of these many potential adverse effects.

Physicians planning to use steroid therapy should develop a clear list of problems for which they are seeking solutions so that, after the treatment is started, an objective analysis of its success can be made and weighed against the risks of the treatment, since, according to Dr. Kaplan, individuals vary in their ability to tolerate the same doses of steroid medication. The patient can only be a cooperating partner if he or she appreciates the benefits of the treatment objectively as well as subjectively. This understanding also helps put the activity of a disease like lupus in perspective. Steroid therapy must be gradually reduced once it has produced satisfactory results, but the physician's effort must be to maintain the beneficial effects while reducing the chance of adverse effects. As many know, this is often a difficult as well as a delicate task.

Children with lupus face some additional problems with this treat-

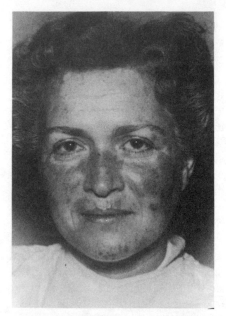

Figure 9a. The butterfly rash appeared on Mrs. Aladjem's cheeks and nose after she had spent time in the sun. The rash is one of many signs that may appear in lupus patients prior to medical therapy.

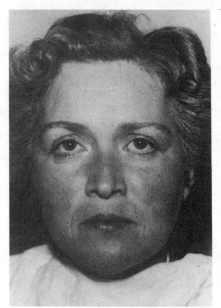

Figure 9b. Mrs. Aladjem developed a "moon face" from steroid therapy.

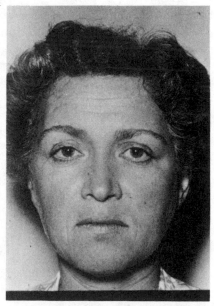

Figure 9c. When the steroid treatment was stopped, the rash disappeared from Mrs. Aladjem's face.

ment, since steroids may affect the rate of growth. If an individual is receiving steroids, the normal potential of the adrenal gland to make cortisone, and be stimulated by ACTH, is suppressed and dulled. This dovetails with the other major reason why an individual who has been receiving steroids for a prolonged period of time must reduce the dosage gradually. Particularly with the lower doses of steroids, according to Dr. Kaplan, a gradual reduction of dosage will permit the adrenal gland to gradually regain its sensitivity to the ACTH, and its normal controlling influences.

How long can patients safely take steroids? Dr. Kaplan stresses that one way to retain many of the beneficial effects of steroids, and reduce some of the unwanted adverse effects, is to provide the treatment over the briefest possible period. As long as the therapeutic benefits can be maintained, the steroid medication should be taken at one time in the morning, rather than spaced out over the day, and taken only every other day. Again, this should be done only with careful and specific directions from the physician, and only if the usefulness of the therapy is retained. Occasionally, however, a physician may decide to eliminate the steroid therapy altogether after a very prolonged period of excellent control of the disease, sometimes several months. This requires an extremely close working relationship between physician and patient, since careful judgments must be made about what to do with minor symptoms that may appear, not as manifestations of SLE, but as a result of reduced dependency on steroid therapy.

In summary, Dr. Kaplan thinks that steroid therapy "is the epitome of the double-edged sword image of medical treatment, even when it is life-saving. It should be used for those manifestations of lupus that must be controlled and that cannot be treated adequately by other less potent means. Clinical researchers are trying to document the circumstances when steroid therapy is most helpful and appropriate, and to develop newer compounds that will achieve the antiinflammatory effects without the potential for adverse effects. In addition, in recent years investigators have been attempting to discover new dosage regimens using the corticosteroids that may be effective in controlling lupus activity but that produce fewer of the unwanted side effects. One dosage regiment in current use is pulse therapy, in which very large single doses of corticosteroids are administered intravenously for three consecutive days. This type of program is considered most often when the patient's condition appears to be deteriorating in spite of significant daily doses of corticosteroids and/or other medications used for the treatment of SLE. While pulse therapy does seem to avoid the long-term adverse effects of steroids, such as the loss of calcium from bone and the redistribution of the fatty tissues, it is not totally free of associated problems. Following such therapy with corticosteroids, some patients have developed seizures or serious bacterial infections."

Dr. Ronald V. Carr of Dalhousie University has conducted numerous studies of SLE patients who are being given alternate-day steroids. Such a regimen was previously felt to be relatively ineffective in treating SLE, although presumably safer than daily therapy because it would produce fewer side effects.

According to Dr. Carr, physicians have been interested in the possibility that, at least in some patients with SLE, alternate-day steroids might be effective. Researchers have now found that in certain patients, whose dosage is followed by frequent visits and laboratory testing, alternate-day steroid therapy can be effective. These studies are still inconclusive, and the long-term effects of such a treatment regimen are now being assessed. It cannot yet be advised as a routine approach to treatment, but preliminary studies do look promising. Eventually, Dr. Carr hopes, carefully selected patients with lupus can be treated in this way.

Nonsteroidal Antiinflammatory Drugs (NSAIDs)

One group of widely used drugs that suppress inflammation is unrelated to any form of cortisone and therefore is referred to as the nonsteroidal antiinflammatory drugs (NSAID). NSAIDs can be further divided into smaller groups depending on their chemical structures. One group, salicylates, includes the most widely known and used NSAID, aspirin. Despite a wide range of newer potent prescription drugs, aspirin remains the treatment of choice to counter some of the painful inflammation caused by lupus in many patients, not only because aspirin is so effective, but also because it can be taken by most people day in and day out for a long time without serious ill effects.

In order for aspirin to be effective, it must be taken regularly, usually four times a day or approximately every four waking hours, so that a certain level of the drug is maintained in the bloodstream.

All drugs are changed and gradually eliminated by chemical systems in the body, so that if one takes the medication sporadically, the level of the drug that is required for its antiinflammatory effect is rarely obtained, and no improvement can be expected. This is an important difference, therefore, from just taking a couple of aspirin to alleviate an annoying pain or headache. It is also important to know, especially with aspirin, that when antiinflammatory doses of the drug are being used, increasing the dosage must be done very gradually, and the new blood level and improvement may not occur for four to five days after raising the dosage. Aspirin as a NSAID has been used to treat some limited manifestations of inflammation in lupus, such as arthritis.

Aspirin does have side effects. According to Dr. Kaplan, some, but by no means all, patients with lupus who receive aspirin regularly may develop changes in their liver tissue that produce abnormalities in the blood tests that are used to measure liver function. For this reason, some physicians substitute other NSAIDs, which were developed primarily for use in other rheumatic disorders. Other, more generally known adverse effects can result from treatment with aspirin, such as gastrointestinal distress. Occasionally, gastrointestinal distress from taking aspirin can lead to an ulcer of the stomach wall. The minor gastrointestinal symptoms can sometimes be avoided by always taking the medication right after meals, with a large glass of water, and using special preparations with substantial amounts of a buffering agent in the same tablet or preparations of coated aspirin that will not dissolve until they pass through the stomach. Most widely advertised over-the-counter preparations are mainly aspirin. Some preparations, whose names suggest they contain added buffers to the aspirin, do not have buffering strength sufficient to make a difference to those who must take large quantities of pills daily. Other widely advertised over-the-counter preparations that do not contain aspirin or any other salicylate usually contain acetominophen (e.g., Tylenol). Acetominophen is less likely to irritate the stomach, but has little or none of the antiinflammatory activity that aspirin or other NSAIDs provide.

Aspirin can also cause other common side effects, including adverse effects on the nervous system. An early sign of this effect is a buzzing sound (called tinnitus) heard by the patient. This harmless effect can be eliminated by decreasing the dosage and thus avoiding the possibility of more serious side effects on the nervous system. Older individuals who may lack the ability to hear this early warning sign should receive special care and monitoring for adverse effects, such as a change in personality, when they are on an aspirin program.

Aspirin also affects the normal functioning of an important factor in blood clotting, the platelets, and should be avoided when the effects of SLE or the use of other drugs decrease the blood's ability to clot properly.

In recent years, clinicians have also become aware of the potential of aspirin and other NSAIDs to affect kidney function. This is more likely to be a problem when an individual has a significant disease, like SLE, already affecting the kidneys. When the kidneys are being stressed because of a systemic illness or are the site of inflammation, they become more dependent on their ability to make chemicals called prostaglandins, which help to maintain the proper blood flow to the kidneys. Aspirin and the other NSAIDs may block the ability of the kidney tissue to make the prostaglandins and thus worsen the kidney function. Although worsening of the kidney function does not occur frequently when lupus patients receive aspirin and other NSAIDs, kidney function should be monitored regularly and is of particular concern when a flareup of lupus activity occurs and the conditions of stressed and/or inflamed kidneys prevail.

Dr. Kaplan emphasizes that despite all these concerns, aspirin still remains a very inexpensive and potentially effective medication for dealing with some forms of inflammation in SLE. Also, a dose of two aspirin, taken occasionally to alleviate a headache or a minor pain, is still one of the best bargains in health care for most people, including individuals with SLE.

Recently, some new types of salicylates, such as choline magnesium salicylate (Trilisate) have been introduced into medical practice. According to Dr. Kaplan, these drugs are said to produce fewer adverse effects on the stomach, and, because they stay in the bloodstream longer, fewer pills must be taken in order to maintain the antiinflammatory level in the blood. However, they are much more expensive than aspirin, and they can be obtained only by prescription since the dosage must be carefully controlled. The level of this drug must not be allowed to build up to a point where serious side effects on the nervous system and the metabolic status of the individual can occur. The experience with these newer forms of salicylate is still very limited in patients with SLE. Effects on metabolism with high blood levels of salicylate are especially dangerous for children and the elderly, Dr. Kaplan emphasizes, and people with SLE taking any salicylate regularly must be extremely careful to keep this medication away from children.

The second group of NSAIDs includes a drug called indomethacin (Indocin), which has been available for a number of years, and newer medications of somewhat similar structure, tolectin and sulindac (Clinoril). A third group of available NSAIDs includes three medications called ibuprofen (Motrin, Rufen), fenoprofen calcium (Nalfon), and naproxen (Naprosen). Additional NSAIDs derived from other classes of similar kinds of compounds introduced into medical practice in recent years include meclofenamate sodium (Meclomen) and piroxicam (Feldene). Diflunisal (Dolobid) is also a relatively new NSAID; it is related to the salicylate drugs and was introduced primarily as an analgesic or painkiller. All the NSAIDs, in fact, have painkilling properties that are independent of their antiinflammatory effect. What is important for patients to be aware of is that the analgesic or painkilling dosage is always lower than the antiinflammatory dosage. In other words, if a person is already receiving one of these drugs for lupus inflammation at the appropriate dosage level, increasing the dosage is not likely to relieve further pain, but may increase the likelihood of an undesirable side effect. Also, if a patient is given a pain pill for a dental extraction or some other reason, and is already taking a NSAID regularly for lupus, the additional pain pill should not be another NSAID. Any of these drugs might be used for minimal or moderate inflammation of the joints as manifestations of SLE. Individuals vary widely as to which medication will successfully control this inflammation and be well tolerated. Each medication must be taken regularly, at a proper dosage, in order to maintain the desired level in the body; and they are, of course, never interchangeable.

NSAIDs can work fairly rapidly compared to some other drugs. The patient may use the NSAIDs for three or four weeks before experiencing the full benefit. Several of the medications, including sulindac, naproxen, piroxicam, and diflunisal, normally stay longer in the body and, therefore, require fewer daily doses to have an antiinflammatory effect. All these medications are relatively expensive, however, and this should be a consideration.

It is important to note that all these medications can cause gastrointestinal problems. Other possible adverse effects include mild dizziness and blurring of vision. Indomethacin produces a particularly high incidence of morning headaches, or a dulling of the senses and forgetfulness. Meclofenamate sodium can produce diarrhea. An adverse effect that has been specifically identified in lupus patients who take ibuprofen has been the occasional development of headache, malaise, and neck pain indicative of an aseptic meningitis (an *extremely* rare complication). If a patient is truly allergic to aspirin, experiences a hivelike rash referred to as urticaria, or develops wheezing, he or she may have this same reaction when any other NSAID is prescribed. This seems to occur more severely in patients who have a history of many allergies, and who have—or had—nasal polyps. The worsening of kidney function that may occur with aspirin therapy when the kidneys are inflamed or stressed because of systemic disease activity may also develop when the individual takes any of the other NSAIDs. The use of any of these drugs may also result in fluid retention, as well as the common types of allergic reactions that can occur with any medication. In fact, there is no extensive well-documented experience with any of these drugs in large numbers of patients with SLE, although they are used, with some success, in selected clinical situations with the rheumatic manifestations of lupus.

According to Dr. Kaplan, the best source of information about the proper use of and precautions for all medications is the *Dispensing Information—Advice for the Patient* book published by the U.S. Pharmacopiae, which uses panels of experts to organize thoughtfully information about each drug for patients.

Anti-malarial drugs

Hydroxychloroquine (Plaquenil), an altogether different type of medication, is also widely used in the treatment of SLE. It is related to a group of compounds first found to be useful in treating malaria, and then discovered to have unique antiinflammatory properties of their own. While other members of this family of drugs are occasionally used in treating SLE, hydroxychloroquine is the most widely prescribed. It has been found effective in controlling some of the inflammation and, in particular, many of the skin manifestations of SLE.

Although it occurs rarely, according to Dr. Kaplan, one of the more serious adverse effects of antimalarial drugs is the tendency of these medications to accumulate in the pigmented tissues in the retina of the eye, which may very seldomly result in blindness. This is definitely related to the total dose of the medication taken over a period of time, thus the recommended dosage of this drug should not be exceeded. Deposits in the lens of the eye may also occur, and an early sign of that problem is when the individual taking the drug complains about seeing halos about street lights or lamps. These symptoms disappear if the drug is reduced or stopped, and is independent of the potential problem of the drug accumulating in the retina. If a patient benefits from this drug and continues to use it, he or she should have a careful eye examination every six months by an ophthalmologist acquainted with the drug's toxicity. Other side effects may include gastrointestinal distress, skin rashes, and occasionally weakness of the muscles or decreased hearing acuity. However, most individuals taking any one of these medications, and using proper and adequate dosages, do not experience any of the adverse effects. Hydroxychloroquine can be very effective in selected problems in lupus patients, but it does take effect slowly. Improvement seldom occurs before a month, and three to six months may pass before the maximum benefit is noted.

Cytotoxic Drugs

Some medications have been adopted for use in SLE not because of any potential to suppress inflammation directly, but because of their ability to affect the cells of the immune systems. Since a basic cause of the inflammation and injury to tissues and organs that we call SLE is a disturbance in the proper functioning of the immune system, these drugs are targeted at this system.

According to Dr. Kaplan, medical researchers do not as yet understand all they need to know about the factors producing this kind of disturbance, although they are the object of a good deal of current research. "When drugs were developed to treat malignant diseases, they were designed to injure cells fatally, with the hope that the tumor cells would be more sensitive than the normal cells of the body. Researchers soon noted that the cells of the immune system, the lymphocytes, were particularly susceptible to some of these medications, and the ability of the immune system to function was altered. When it was observed that the function of the immune system might be suppressed by these compounds, they were tested in patients with very severe forms of disorders like SLE, where the immune system appeared to be abnormal and contributing to the disease process. In one specific situation (controlling the immune system after a kidney transplantation), these drugs have proven necessary for satisfactory results. Over the years, two medications, so-called cytotoxic (cell-killing) drugs, have been used with variable success both in patients with severe SLE unresponsive to other treatment and in those patients requiring unacceptably high doses of steroids. One of these drugs is azathioprine (Imuran), and the other is cyclophosphamide (Cytoxan, Neosan). The use of these drugs with SLE patients who have serious kidney involvement remains one of the most-dicussed issues among physicians with expertise in treating lupus. Some physicians think that these patients will tend to do at least as well by being on one of these medications, and lower doses of steroids, rather than on higher doses of steroids alone.

"While cytotoxic drugs do produce side effects, they are not the same effects; thus, the incidence and seriousness of the side effects from the overall treatment can be reduced using this approach. Because cytotoxic drugs can affect the normal, rapidly dividing cells in the bone marrow, the blood counts of lupus patients taking them must be carefully monitored. As is true with all medications, and particularly with these drugs, the prescribing of drugs and the proper monitoring of their use is a serious contractual arrangement between physician and patient. The patient not only has the right to be well informed about medication, but he or she must also understand and be committed to the monitoring procedures needed to make sure that the medication can be administered as safely as possible."

In addition to its effects in the blood count, azathioprine sometimes produces other adverse effects when it is first administered, including an effect on the liver, or gastrointestinal distress. The dose may be reduced if an individual has preexisting liver disease, or is taking a drug called allopurinal to reduce uric acid. In such cases, the dosage of azathioprine must be very greatly reduced, and the patient's blood tests must be followed with great care. Cyclophosphamide, which some people feel may be preferable to azathioprine in similar circumstances, must also be given with extreme care and close monitoring. In addition to serious effects on the blood count and occasional gastrointestinal distress, regular usage may cause the hair to fall out, although this is generally reversible. Another potential problem, according to Dr. Kaplan, is the tendency of the drug to produce bladder irritation; people with relatively normal kidney function who are taking cyclophosphamide are encouraged to drink ten to twelve extra glasses of water each day so that the irritating breakdown products of cyclophosphamide will not concentrate in the bladder.

Unfortunately, long-term complications with cyclophosphamide are possible, although not very common. According to Dr. Kaplan, "These include scarring of the bladder, and sterility, which may not be reversible. Another concern with these cytotoxic drugs are other effects on the genetic material of the body. Although the delivery of normal babies has been recorded among parents who were taking a drug like azathioprine, physicians are concerned about the development *in utero* of a fetus conceived and maturing while a parent was taking one of these cytotoxic drugs. In addition, there is reason to believe that individuals taking these medications may face an increased risk of developing certain malignancies later in life. While this risk has not been established for patients with SLE, information from other types of patients raise this as at least a theoretical possibility for the SLE patient receiving azathioprine or cyclophosphamide.

"Because of these potential long-term effects and known short-term effects, these drugs should be considered for use with SLE only in the severest form of the disease, and in an attempt to evade other unacceptable adverse effects from high doses of steroids. Advances in an understanding of the metabolism of lymphocytes has recently led researchers to work toward the development of new types of agents that may manipulate the immune system in a manner more specific than is possible with currently available drugs. As we learn more about these drugs, we hope they will be looked at with regard to the serious problem of SLE."

Drug-induced Lupus
The pharmaceutical profession has been very successful in making new drugs for the treatment of lupus in the past few decades. When such drugs are available, doctors will prescribe them and patients will use them. Some doctors, however, are concerned about the widespread use of over-the-counter drugs. Such self-dosage of a variety of medications, many of them unknown to the physician,

can cause serious problems. According to Dr. Kaplan, "Sulfa-type drugs are among those most clearly implicated in the exacerbation of lupus. That is why, when treating a urinary tract infection in anyone with lupus, physicians should use nonsulfa antibiotics. Many other drugs, including diuretics and dyes given for radiographic studies, have also been found, in isolated circumstances, to exacerbate the symptoms of true lupus. However, even though a drug such as penicillin has been implicated in this way, its use in the patient with lupus may still be considered if the particular infection is best treated by that particular drug. Physicians should, however, be very cautious about administering any medication casually to any patient with lupus.

"Some drugs, including some commonly used medications, may produce signs and symptoms we commonly associate with active systemic lupus erythematosus. This unfortunate development is totally unrelated, as far as we know, to any potential to develop true lupus. In some circumstances these drugs have been used by patients with true lupus, and did not appear to cause any difficulties or worsen the problems of those patients. One of the first of these drugs known to produce a lupuslike drug reaction was hydralazine, when it was being used in fairly high doses for the treatment of hypertension. The studies of the lupuslike reaction with this drug are fairly old, since the higher dosages of hydralazine associated with producing the reaction are generally no longer used.

"The reports in the medical literature indicate that, in addition to antinuclear antibodies, some patients who develop this lupuslike reaction may be found to have anti-DNA antibodies, although this finding is controversial. Low levels of complement are unusual, and it is difficult to evaluate the rare patients who were said to develop some findings of renal disease. Clearly, the development of renal disease is extremely rare in any drug-induced lupus syndromes. One of the most widely used drugs that may produce the lupuslike drug reaction is procainamide, which is used to help control abnormal heart rhythms. Patients receiving procainamide regularly produce antinuclear antibodies, even if they do not get other symptoms of a lupuslike reaction. In fact, if no clinical problems appear, the development of antinuclear antibodies is not considered a sufficient reason to stop the medication when it is needed. Such patients essentially never develop anti-DNA antibodies, low complement levels, or renal disease. They commonly develop joint symptoms and pleurisy, and do develop rashes, although with less frequency than in true lupus. In both these situations, the lupuslike drug reaction clears, generally within weeks, once the offending drug is removed, and, as far as we know, having such a drug reaction is unrelated to any susceptibility for true lupus."

Another widely prescribed drug, isoniazid, which is used in the treatment of tuberculosis, may also induce the development of antinuclear antibodies and, rarely, a lupuslike drug reaction that ceases after the drug is stopped. Older literature also suggests that some effective, commonly used anticonvulsants, such as phenytoin sodium (Dilantin), mephenytoin (Mesantoin), and trimethadione (Tridione), may induce a lupuslike drug reaction; Dr. Kaplan has reviewed these reports and found them confusing and a little anecdotal, based solely on retrospective observations. These reports, however, should probably not alter the use of these drugs with patients who have true lupus, when their use is indicated for central nervous system problems. There is no reason to believe they are at all harmful to the patient with true lupus.

Drugs That Exacerbate Lupus

Certain medications, such as penicillin or tetracycline, may exacerbate lupus symptoms, including fever, joint pains, butterfly rash, and nausea, but this is altogether different from the drug-induced lupus syndrome caused by certain drugs. Antibiotics, however, rarely produce problems in patients with lupus. Therefore, any such reaction to medication in a patient with lupus should be noted by the patient and made known to the physician. But Dr. Kaplan emphasizes the importance of using any medication judiciously and only for clearcut indications in the patient: "Viral infections, such as the common cold and uncomplicated flu, are unaffected by antibiotics, and their casual use in these circumstances adds no benefit and only creates the potential for a complication from the drug itself. On the other hand, infections are often a real problem for the lupus patient, and effective antibiotics may be required to treat them. If any individual with lupus is known to react poorly to any one antibiotic, we are fortunate today to have an impressive array of such drugs to choose from in handling most forms of bacterial infection, and this type of infection must be adequately treated. I do not think any drug 'causes' lupus. Rather, some drugs exacerbate preexisting true lupus, and other drugs, generally different ones, can cause a lupuslike reaction to the drug, a reaction unrelated, as far as we know, to susceptibility to true lupus. Discontinuance of such a drug results in complete clearing of all the signs and symptoms of the syndrome."

Rest and Medication

When I was experiencing active lupus, my Bulgarian doctor, Professor Liuben Popoff, believed that rest was essential in the treatment of lupus. He felt that bed rest, proper nutrition, and peace of mind or emotional rest were important—as important as the persistent use of high doses of corticosteroids. This is most forcefully expressed by Dr. Marion W. Ropes in her book *Systemic Lupus Erythematosus*, published by Harvard University Press in 1976. Dr. Ropes strongly encourages a strict rest period in order to allow a patient to maintain maximum resistance to resurgence of disease activity. In addition, lupus patients are known to be susceptible to infections, and it is important for them to minimize their contacts with sources of infection in individuals outside their home. My own current doctor believes that even when the disease is in remission, the management of lupus must be taken seriously. He believes that lupus patients should have limited work schedules, in some cases limited even to the essential tasks in the care of their home and children, and if possible, they should not work outside their home.

I believe that rest, along with good medical care, has played an important role in my recovery. Some patients have used Transcendental Meditation with success.

Even in remission, I am still "fragile." I fatigue easily, and I am still sensitive to the sun, to cold, to heat, to everything that touches my skin, and I still need lots of rest and lots of sleep to cope with the demands of everyday living.

Through the years, I have learned a great deal about myself and about lupus. I have lost my fear of the disease, as well as my fear of imminent death.

When patients ask me what I am doing to stay well, I tell them that I am a perfect example of Sir William Osler's aphorism: "If you want to live a long life, get a chronic disease and learn how to take care of it."

VITAMIN THERAPY UNDER INVESTIGATION FOR LUPUS

Many lupus patients claim that they have a lower concentration of some vitamins in their bodies than other people, or lower vitamin activity. According to Dr. Ronald V. Carr, associate professor of medicine, department of medicine and department of microbiology at Dalhousie University in Canada, the role of vitamin therapy in various diseases is a major problem. He points out that in vitamin deficiency states, vitamin therapy is the appropriate treatment. Vitamin therapy is advocated by some individuals in response to a variety of diseases, ranging from the common cold to SLE. Said Dr. Carr, "I would not be surprised to find that vitamins are beneficial in certain conditions which, as of now, are not associated with vitamin deficiencies.

"As to the use of vitamin therapy in SLE, a number of lupus patients (and probably some physicians as well) believe that taking vitamin supplements (sometimes in large quantities) has resulted in a marked improvement in their state of well-being." Dr. Carr does not discount the changes such people describe, but points out that a number of factors must be considered before everyone jumps on the vitamin bandwagon. First, lupus is a disease that frequently has spontaneous remissions, which may last for long periods, and drug-induced remissions, which may last just as long in some individuals. If a remission occurs during the time patients are given vitamin therapy, they and their treatment team will probably attribute their getting better to the vitamins, which, in fact, may have absolutely nothing to do with the improvement. Secondly, some of the manifestations of SLE that are an obvious problem to the patient, like fatigue and the feeling of weakness, often have a psychological component as well. If this psychological component is affected by an individual's faith in vitamins, an increase in well-being may certainly occur, and it may be attributed by the person to a biochemical effect of the vitamins.

According to Dr. Carr, a number of years ago physicians thought vitamin B12, pantothenic acid, and vitamin E might have an effect on SLE, but careful studies have failed to support these observations. But, as he points out, some individuals swear by vitamin therapy, even though no scientific evidence supports their impressions. Most physicians believe, at least as of now, that vitamins should be used by people who have vitamin-deficiency diseases, but not as a shotgun therapeutic approach to SLE.

As our knowledge of nutrition grows we may find certain nutritional factors per se that can affect the disease.

7

Lupus and Photosensitivity

I spoke with Dr. Elizabeth Cole, a dermatologist who takes care of many people with lupus, about the sensitivity to sunlight experienced by many of her lupus patients, a sensitivity that implicates ultraviolet radiation as a possible factor in triggering or exacerbating symptoms of the disease. Skin rashes and lesions often appear on the parts of the body exposed to the sun, and a lupus patient's symptoms in general may become aggravated by such exposure.

Dr. Cole is chief of dermatology at Newton-Wellesley Hospital in Newton, Massachusetts, and assistant clinical professor in dermatology, Tufts University School of Medicine, Boston.

According to Dr. Cole, lupus patients are affected by more than just bright sunlight. A great deal of ultraviolet (UV) light also comes through fog and clouds, and much is reflected from ground surfaces, buildings, and plants into shadowed areas. In addition, UV rays are emitted from man-made sources. According to Dr. Cole, the pathogenic role of UV radiation is not entirely understood. Ultraviolet radiation is thought to enhance the immune response and disrupt the natural tolerance to DNA. Lupus skin lesions or systemic illness may follow other noxious stimuli, including thermal burns and insect bites; sunburn may act as a nonspecific trauma to cells. Specific antibodies to UV-altered DNA can be induced in experimental animals with exposure to UV radiation. Some researchers have proposed that patients with lupus are immunized to UV-altered DNA, and that the antibodies subsequently produced in their bodies cross-react with the DNA of their own living cells.

One third to one half of all patients with lupus are overtly photosensitive. Said Dr. Cole, "We cannot know the real number of photosensitive lupus patients unless we could prevent all exposure to potentially dangerous radiation. That sunburn can precipitate or exacerbate SLE, with or without skin changes, is well recognized. In one laboratory experiment, patients with lupus who were exposed to solar and artificial UV light developed lesions. These lesions lasted for many months following the exposure. Lupus patients can sometimes react to even small amounts of radiation in UV-A and UV-B ranges."

UV-B is the classification given to those rays that cause sunburn and tanning reaction, with wavelengths in the range of 290 to 320 nanometers (a nanometer is a very small measurement of length, one-billionth of a meter, used to measure X-ray waves, ultraviolet light, visible light, and infrared). UV-A includes those rays that cause immediate tanning of the skin, with wavelengths in the range of 320 to 400 nanometers (nm).

Despite my remission, I told Dr. Cole, I develop a burning sensation on my face when I use the photostatting machine, and I become unduly tired as if I were going to become ill again.

Dr. Cole explained that the light source I had been exposed to emits visible light (wavelengths 400–760 nm) that normally does not harm a lupus patient, but it also has some UV-A waves that cannot be seen and are of lengths to which some people may be sensitive.

"You probably wouldn't feel ill from a very short time at the machine, but the more flashes, the more exposure to ultraviolet radiation. Actually, you are very close to the light source when you use the machine. The distance from the source of radiation, and the length of time of exposure, are as important to you as the wavelength. It is very important to realize that sources of UV-A and UV-B radiation are encountered frequently, the most common being fluorescent and high-intensity light bulbs. Many very different types of fluorescent light bulbs are manufactured, but not all of them emit ultraviolet waves. Unfortunately, in a public place, one doesn't have control over what types are used. For instance, if you have a single fluorescent light emitting some ultraviolet waves in your kitchen or bathroom, you might or might not be bothered by it, because photosensitivity varies from one individual to another. Also, different wavelengths are produced by different types of light bulbs. However, if you have lupus, and are a draftsman, for instance, or work in an office where banks of fluorescent bulbs line the ceiling, and perhaps also have a high-intensity bulb on your desk, you might spend eight to ten hours a day with intensive, even relatively distant exposure, and be made very sick by it. Other patients with lupus might not be bothered at all. It is quite an individual matter. Tolerance to UV light in a lupus patient tends to remain stable, but I have seen cases where it changed dramatically and suddenly."

Thus it is important to know what specific radiation sources are potentially harmful to SLE patients to prevent exacerbations. Although most photosensitive lupus patients are sensitive to the UV-B range, some patients are sensitive to UV-A. These waves go through glass; when you are seated on the sunny side of a plane at 35,000 feet, you are exposed to a lot of UV-A if you are not protected. Dr. Cole stresses that anyone on a glass porch or in a car, without a UV-A protective light screen, is being exposed to visible radiation and UV-A as well.

Incandescent light bulbs produce no significant UV-A or UV-B—although they do give off lots of visible light and some infrared energy, which is felt as heat. Visible light will do no harm, but, of course, infrared can produce a thermal burn.

Lupus patients should also be aware of other sources of UV-A or UV-B. Welders' arcs produce a great deal of UV-A and UV-B, depending on the amount of heat produced. Tungsten iodide light sources, such as are used in movie or slide projectors, radiate lots of UV-A, and so do the hot furnaces of the steel industry. A moviehouse projectionist or a teacher who uses films might have problems if unprotected.

A burning fire or surgical lights do not emit UV-A or UV-B, but surgical lights can injure the lupus patient, because of the emission of a different kind of UV light, UV-C (200–290 nm). And, of course, X-ray radiation is damaging, and no topical protection is possible for that. The high-intensity lights used in photographic, TV, and other studios might also have UV-A emission. Color televisions may also have an adverse effect on photosensitive lupus patients.

According to Dr. Cole, until two to four years ago, very little attention was paid to the amount of UV emission that came from TV sets to viewers' bodies. Since then, however, an effort has been made to change the screen's design to eliminate ultraviolet emission.

Here again, the length of time of exposure is important; four to six hours in front of an older UV-emitting screen definitely could harm an SLE patient. I myself have developed bluish spots on my face after appearing on TV talk shows, which use very high-intensity lighting.

It is essential for lupus patients to be particularly careful about their exposure to the sun—always. Recently I developed two new spots on my cheeks after I was in the sun for half an hour waiting for a taxi. Dr. Cole explained that the damage had been done very innocently. Lupus patients must train themselves to use light screens, the way others take pills for their illnesses. This can be difficult. Sunscreens are an important protection. Sunscreens consist of UV photosensitive chemicals held in suspension in a vehicle that can be applied to the skin. These chemicals can bond to the skin and act as a trap for the UV energy that strikes the skin. They do this by reflecting and absorbing the energy in its own molecules. No sunscreen is perfect, and some energy does go through, penetrating into the skin. Sunscreens differ tremendously in their effectiveness, even when the ingredient looks the same and the SPF (sun protection factor) reads the same.

Not all doctors are aware of the importance of sunscreen protection for lupus patients. Said Dr. Cole, "The science of clinical photobiology is new, developed during the past decade; although its body of data is widely published, it is largely found in journals directed toward dermatologists, rather than internists or other physicians who deal with lupus patients. I believe that dermatologists, who once played an important role in the diagnosis and treatment of lupus patients, should be brought back into the teamwork care of the lupus patient. We have a lot of knowledge and skills to help the patient and perhaps prevent scarring if we are consulted early enough. Irreversible scars can occur as early as four to six weeks after the onset of a lesion of the skin.

"None of the sunscreens available require prescription, but it's important for lupus patients to be careful in their selection. The sunscreen industry makes products they want to sell to as many people as possible. They tend to cater to the person who 'wants a little color,' and that is not good enough for most lupus patients. Only recently have physicians become aware that many people have limited tolerance to ultraviolet light, for serious medical reasons.

Doctors need education, too, about which agents shut out which UV radiation sufficiently to protect lupus patients."

Dr. Cole emphasizes how important it is for every lupus patient, light-sensitive or not, to be protected with *daily* use of the most potent available UV-A *and* UV-B-blocking agents. Lupus patients seldom need to wear two lotions, since combined potent UV-A and UV-B protection has become more available. All light blockers except the opaque ones are easily washed off, however, and actually disappear from the skin in a short time (about ninety minutes) out of doors and after swimming or sweating. "One can easily forget that," Dr. Cole said, "so carry your lotion with you at all times."

Dr. Cole prefers to call the light screens "blocking agents" in order to emphasize that visible light is not the enemy: "Many light screens or suntan lotions are on the market, but most of them are for normal people, and they really are not very effective. At present there are five chemical classes of protective agents. The chemical structures of these substances have a special affinity for only certain wavelengths of UV light. They are: Para-aminobenzoic acid (PABA), which guards against UV-B, as do cinnamates, homo-methyl salicylate, and anthranilate, the latter two of which are too weak when used alone to be of much use to lupus patients; and benzophenones, which guard against UV-A and UV-B. The important thing to know is that the vehicle into which one or more of these chemicals is put can modify its efficacy. In other words, even the most effective chemical used to block UV absorption can be rendered useless to a lupus patient, or other person who needs a sunscreen for medical reasons, by the presence of other combined chemicals, such as certain emollients, which destroy its activity. Sweat, water, evaporation, and ambient humidity may also reduce the effectiveness of sunscreens. There are also opaque screens, which put a visible physical barrier in the way. They are probably the most effective blocking agents we have. However, they are not as cosmetically acceptable to some people. The best-tinted ones are: Continuous Coverage by Clinique, Reflecta, and Covermark. Those would be ideal for time spent under strong UV-emitting lights, or any time when the patient wants to have makeup on and still be safe. The untinted stark white opaque screens are titanium dioxide and zinc oxide."

Several very recent studies allow researchers to rank sun-blocking agents by number, in order of their protective ability (SPF), 15 and above being the most protective. The designation SPF as used on labels by the industry is not always standard. In fact, the European products, such as Piz Buin, are numbered differently (in Europe 8 is equal to an American 15). UV-A and UV-B blockers are together in the same gel, cream or lotion, one that has been specially selected to provide maximum efficacy. It is extremely important to realize that not all screens labeled with an SPF of 15 are equal where it counts—in real-life situations such as sweaty sports, gardening, and swimming. Some well-known, popular, and highly recommended blockers with an SPF of 15 actually fall to an SPF of 2 after brief exposure to sweat or water. "At this time," Dr. Cole said, "the best sunscreens for lupus patients are: Ti Screen 15, and Piz Buin cream or lotion with SPF of 12. These two do not contain PABA but do contain benzophenone and cinnamate. Of those containing PABA and benzophenone, the best are Sundown 15, MMM What-A-Tan, Total Eclipse 15, Coppertone's Supershade, and Presun 15 (creamy lotion). Patients can develop contact dermatitis to any of the active or vehicle ingredients, but especially from PABA. Then they cannot use screens containing the allergen, but must use other types. They should consult a dermatologist, who will help them figure out what they can use. Sometimes this contact dermatitis needs light to develop." Dr. Cole explained that cross-reactions can also occur, and individuals allergic to phenothiazide and sulfonamide drugs or hair dyes cannot use PABA without developing a rash. In this case patients can use Ti Screen or Piz Buin 12, which contain benzophenone and cinnamate, or those products containing benzophenone alone.

As for screening the scalp from the sun, Dr. Cole pointed out that hair itself is some protection, although in lupus patients it is often thin. A hat provides good protection, but hats are not sufficient protection for the face and arms because radiation is reflected from sand, concrete, and other surfaces. Of course, the protection provided by hats, like all clothing, depends on the tightness of weave. "I'm not sure people realize that a see-through blouse is almost no protection at all," Dr. Cole said.

According to Dr. Cole, there is an area of disagreement among physicians when it comes to warning lupus patients to be more careful about avoiding the various types of radiation: "I know some will feel I am coming on way too strong about the role of light in lupus. But I do not know beforehand, nor do I have a satisfactory way of testing to find out, who will get new skin lesions, or who may feel or become systemically ill from ultraviolet light from any source. We know of no safe way to test. A lupus patient who is usually not sensitive can become sensitive without warning. One patient in particular comes to mind. She was a very pretty young girl with barely visible lesions. Her skin biopsy was positive for lupus, and her minimal lab tests indicated asymptomatic systemic lupus. For a long time she was very careful to use blocking agents, but she slipped up just one afternoon at a flea market. She came back to me many weeks after these new lesions first appeared. We have been struggling to clear her of these lesions for the past two years, but, I'm sorry to say, they will be scarring forever. I am so sorry she did not let me know soon enough to help prevent the scars." The patient also developed joint pains and a disfiguring rash from just one day of too much UV light. "The main idea is to keep informing both patients and physicians," Dr. Cole said. Lupus patients need to wear an effective screen every single day, whether they are indoors or out, whether they are in the shade or in direct light, and they should let their physicians know immediately if a skin lesion appears, so that treatment can start right away. "Even if you feel like you have a lot of sunscreen on, don't take any chances," Dr. Cole said. "It is not worth it." Wearing UV radiation screens is like buying insurance. You never know when you might need it. Only recently has she advised such universal use of screening in lupus patients. Many lupus patients have had to learn the hard way. Even though all patients are not obviously photosensitive, Dr. Cole believes they would all be wise to protect themselves. Those who are not light-sensitive, she said, can then go about indoors or outdoors, in the sun or shade, with a greater feeling of safety. A few patients who are exquisitely sensitive, even with the best current screens, may still not be safe in the hours of intense sun radiation, 9 A.M. to 4 P.M.

The seasons of the year or the latitude also make a difference in the amount of UV light present. In New England, the sun is intense enough to damage between March 15 and October 15, but further toward the equator, the sun is always dangerous. This is because the distance traveled in the ozone layer affects the amount of radiation reaching earth from the sun, and varies with the seasons, as well as with the time of day.

Radiation is also reflected from surfaces such as water, snow, and sand, just as visible light is reflected from a mirror. There is a lot of UV light around, even on a cloudy day. At such times the lupus patient must realize that he or she is exposed, not only to incident radiation, but also to light reflecting from the other surfaces. Dr. Cole said, "I certainly do not want to create neuroses in any patients, especially lupus patients, about light. But I strongly believe that until we understand exactly how one lupus patient is photosensitive, we cannot afford to ignore the importance of UV radiation for all lupus patients. Lupus patients have nothing to lose by knowing the rules of radiation, where it is, and how to protect themselves from it, and then doing it without fail.

"There are other advantages of using potent sunscreens. Wrinkles and some of the other signs of aging, including solar keratoses and skin cancers, are also caused by UV light."

I also interviewed Dr. Madhu A. Pathak at Massachusetts General Hospital in Boston about lupus and photosensitivity. Dr. Pathak is senior associate in dermatology (biochemistry) at Harvard University Medical School. Dr. Pathak is in agreement with Dr. Cole: "A number of factors are known to induce the appearance of skin lesions in chronic lupus patients. The agent most often incriminated is sunlight. Also, exposure to radiation from artificial light sources, such as the high-intensity fluorescent bulbs, can exacerbate the disease. The lesions of some patients also appear to become worse with infrared radiation, such as that from electric heaters. Patients develop skin lesions with the onset of hot weather or under the influence of cold and wind.

"The role of immune complexes in the pathogenesis of lupus is well recognized. The patient should know that UV radiation causes specific chemical transformation in the genetic material of the skin, the DNA molecules. This UV-altered DNA is antigenic. We know that sera of patients with systemic lupus react with UV-altered DNA. This UV-altered material, when released in the circulation, can lead to the induction of antibodies directed against skin or other tissues.

"Thus, to avoid this possibility, the most important measure the patient can take is to avoid sun exposure. However, in daily life, one cannot avoid exposure to sunlight. He or she must, therefore, resort to regular use of effective sunscreen creams and lotions. The face, the neck, any exposed area of the chest, the arms, and the hands should be shielded with effective sunscreens that have sun protection value of 15 or more. He or she should know that sweating, swimming, or washing removes the protective film of the sunscreen. The sunscreen, therefore, must be reapplied."

Researchers are trying to develop a systemic sunscreen that, when taken orally by lupus patients once a day, would be distributed evenly in the skin and provide day-long protection to the DNA molecules of the skin. They hope that in the near future research will enable physicians to prescribe such an oral sunscreen.

8

The Patient, the Physician, and the Psychiatrist: Managing The Psychosocial Aspects of Lupus

The past few decades have been an exciting time for research in immunology and lupus, and from the physician's point of view many things have improved. From the patient's point of view, however, these signs of medical progress are not enough. Lupus patients need better diagnostic tests, medications with fewer side effects, and more public awareness of the disease, as well as adequate health insurance and Social Security Disability for patients who need them.

For lupus patients, the disorder remains a bizarre, cruel disease of unknown cause, with an unpredictable prognosis and symptoms that are difficult to explain. Lupus is intermittent, recurrent, and can destroy, in those afflicted by it, both the will to live and the ability to cope. Lupus can threaten life and prevent functioning as a normal human being. But do physicians understand what this disease does to a human life? Without knowing this, can they properly treat their patients? In lupus, the body and the soul are enmeshed in a web of pain and desperation, and, through it all, many patients say they can find no one who understands, no one willing to listen.

Despite the growing awareness of lupus, the disease can still be a lonely experience. Many patients still go from one doctor to another, only to be told that they suffer from a recurring cold or a lingering virus. Some patients are told that the disease exists only in their minds, since they could not have so many unrelated symptoms. And although lupus is known not to be contagious, some patients have even been asked by their physician, "Where did you catch it?" In their search for understanding, some patients become confused and emotionally distraught, even questioning their own sanity.

I have spent many hours at medical libraries searching for information about the psychosocial and emotional problems of lupus patients. I have found very few papers on the subject. Most articles on lupus in psychiatric literature focus on medical aspects of systemic lupus erythematosus with central nervous system involvement. I found nothing on the human story of the lupus patient, either from the patient's point of view or from that of the physician. I found nothing to reflect the fears and apprehensions of the individual, the very core of the disease. Patients outline with great vividness the consequences of chronic illness and particularly of a disease like lupus, which is misunderstood by patients as well as physicians.

One patient wrote:

> My sensitivity to the sun is just one facet of the enigmatic and frustrating disease I have had for thirty years, most of them without knowing it. I have endured months of unnecessary penicillin shots for a venereal disease I never had. Doctors in the past have called me neurotic because I had such a bewildering array of symptoms—skin rashes, joint swellings, aches and pains.

When I spoke with this patient, she said: "My mother died before I was properly diagnosed as having systemic lupus erythematosus. She died thinking that my father was responsible for my so-called venereal disease."

Another patient wrote:

> My husband left me because he was afraid of catching my lupus. He stopped kissing me and went to sleep in a separate room. Once, when he developed an allergic rash on his chest, he went from doctor to doctor convinced that he had lupus, and he blamed me for his problems. My hairdresser

feels like that, too. The last time I went to have my hair washed, he told me not to come back because the other customers were afraid of catching my rashes.

Another patient wrote:

Attached is a copy of an article I came across at the hospital where I work, which states, "Lupus, mostly because of more permissive sexual mores, is probably the fastest increasing disease in the US. [It is] generally if not always transmitted by intercourse." I have been found to have lupus, and this article has me very upset. I took the article to my physician, who informed me it has no basis in fact. He stated that lupus is akin to arthritis, and is an inflammatory disease that causes a breakdown of connective tissue, and in no way has anything to do with intercourse, or sex. . . . Have I been misinformed? Since this paper is one a great many hospitals in Montana subscribe to, I cannot see its value, if the information it contains is incorrect.

A professor of literature at a midwestern university wrote:

People think of me as a hypochondriac, which makes me extremely self-conscious about discussing my lupus problems with anyone. My husband cannot possibly understand, as I don't know enough to explain to him about my illness.

In another letter, she said:

I am frustrated by labels such as "possible collagen disease" and "90 percent chance of lupus." I do not blame my physician for not providing me with a convenient label for my disease. I blame him for not entering into an active struggle with me to search for such a label. . . . No one would believe me at this time. Even my husband thought my vague complaints the product of a distorted and overly sensitive imagination, and what else could he think? The medical profession had "proven" that there was nothing wrong with me. They had labeled me a neurotic. I began to perceive myself as one. I still suffer from the destructive professional attitude of the physicians during these years. I needed so much to define my problems or at least to have someone grope for a definition with me. The medical profession had defined my complaints this way; in the presence of mystery, I had nothing better to offer.

These words were written by a professor of theology:

One thing that hurts me is that many people avoid me out of fear. People feel threatened. I noticed, for instance, when I broke two ribs, that everyone would inquire about them and ask if they could help. They were much more solicitous about the ribs than they were when I got my diagnosis of lupus.

A patient with central nervous system involvement wrote:

I barely manage by an effort of will to keep from speaking, which to me means screaming and crying all day long. Even at night I cannot rest or relax. I find it hard to sleep; then I wake up abruptly and every time I want to go back to sleep I see bright flashes of light. . . . I am losing my memory and sometimes even my judgment. I do things and I don't remember them. . . . I tell people things I don't remember telling them. Like Flannery O'Connor's* heroes, I am constantly judged and accused of crimes I don't remember.

Another problem with lupus is that friends and family see you looking well one moment and distressed the next. They begin to wonder whether you are a hypochondriac or, even worse, a person who is no longer productive, someone who can no longer be depended on. Dr. Naomi Rothfield, a professor of medicine at the University of Connecticut School of Medicine, stresses that patients need understanding from both physician and family. She says the impact of the disease on the patient's physical and mental status is immense, and without the full understanding of the family, the patient flounders. In her opinion, the patient must understand his or her own disease, and must understand the long- and short-range goals of therapy as well as the type of therapy, its side effects, and

* Flannery O'Connor (1925–1964) died of lupus, and so did her father.

its benefits. In addition, she believes the patient's spouse must learn to understand both the disease and its therapy and must also become fully knowledgeable about their emotional impact on the patient.

Lupus imposes a physical, financial, social, and psychological burden on the family. Medical fees and medications are high, and medical insurance is difficult or even impossible to obtain for many lupus patients. Added to the expenses are lost wages and the frequent inability to obtain Social Security Disability, which creates incredible heartaches. Family outings and social activities must often be canceled because of photosensitivity, fatigue, and other symptoms of the disease.

The families of lupus patients are sometimes caught in the bind of feeling annoyance, anger, and guilt. This creates a vicious circle that leads to much stress and depression. A young woman whose mother died of lupus describes her experience with such an ordeal:

> Perhaps the most anguished part of my childhood in relationship to my mother with lupus can be summarized by "not knowing." This lack of knowledge, lack of awareness, manifested itself constantly as I wondered from day to day what the next one held. "Good days" presaged optimism, "bad ones" were something to get through. But, all the time, the question of how long the good ones would be there, how bad the bad ones would get, made it difficult to plan, or to just assume that life would go on as it always had. And "as it always had" meant with fear that my mother might die at any time, guilt that my actions might contribute to it, anger that my mother was not like all the rest, overprotectiveness so that her comfort would be maximized, confusion because she seemed so healthy, as she never let her appearance symbolize how she felt, and resentment because she was always the center of attention. Though my mother valiantly tried to keep the family life within the realm of normal, I always felt guilty when a birthday party or PTA meeting caused her to tire, disappointment when she could not go, deprived when another went with me instead.
>
> As I grew older and more responsible I became more protective and she became weaker. I became the "chief telephone answerer," I intercepted visitors, I anticipated when a rough day would require an afternoon nap. I under-

stood the words, "My mother is not feeling well today," that I repeated so often. Yet I never quite understood why. Though I had knowledge of the doctors' reports, all I could see was a willful woman who refused to play a sick role, whose beauty and grace spoke to a vitality she wanted to have "with health," but whose restrictions on life's activities seemed capricious. After a while I began to wonder whether she was really sick because the symptoms seemed erratic. Then I felt guilty that I doubted her. I was confused because of the many times the lupus went into remission; I was frightened when it returned. Not knowing what was happening or what would happen, when and why, or whether it would even happen again, I spent a lot of time frightened. Nobody else seemed to know, either.

Though I realize that I feel deprived because lupus took something from my childhood, from my family, from my mother, her struggle with it left me with a respect for her that I would not have been forced to develop. Seeing what my mother went through time and time again in the hospitals, knowing that she wanted desperately to be well, watching her give up activities gradually over so many years, and feeling her worry that we should not suffer, left me with a feeling of awe. There were a number of times when I heard doctors say to one another that they could figure out no reason why she was still alive except that she had an incredible will to live—one that kept her alive for over twenty years after she had been informed she had only three more. My mother was a fighter, she waged a war courageously, she lost it with dignity, but she never gave up!

Dr. Theodore Nadelson, Chief of Psychiatry, Boston Veterans Administration and Clinical Professor of Psychiatry, Tufts Medical School, says that one way to gain understanding about the problems of lupus patients is through self-help groups for patients, their families and their physicians. He gives as an example Michael Balint, an English doctor who has started a number of physician groups where doctors talk about their difficulties in dealing with patients (see Chapter 17 for more reading on this subject). Dr. Nadelson says that physicians often avoid reflecting on their own feelings about patients, and seem to do better talking among themselves with a group leader. "We found that such groups are extremely helpful here, but fitting it into a busy practice is, of course, difficult. Doctors simply have to see that this is important," Dr. Nadelson says, "but only some do; the others are hard to convince." Dr. Nadelson points out that lupus patients who have obvious manifestations of disease actually have a much easier time, they do not need to "prove" that they are very ill. Lupus is one of those insidious diseases that produces symptoms before it produces signs. And even when the disease is full-blown, patients may simply feel lousy and not be able to "show anything" to the doctor. Two parallel experiences seem to be occurring—the patients' feelings and subjective impressions of their bodies and themselves, and the physician's way of looking at disease. Dr. Nadelson says that physicians usually view disease in terms of the "body space," and some doctors follow the tenet of the great pathologist, Virchow, who said that where disease occurs, a bodily organ must be affected. If a change in an organ cannot be found at any particular time, then the physician may say no real disease is present. "Of course, our experience in clinical medicine is such that we can only deal with what we know," Dr. Nadelson says. "In other words, we should accept the fact that, when we are ignorant, the symptom the patient describes should be the prevailing one; and we should assume that when patients say they feel tired or have pain, they are tired or in pain. The fact that we cannot find any objective evidence for it in their bodies at the time does not mean that they don't have those two subjective symptoms."

This problem was very well illustrated by the theology professor with two broken ribs that were easier to handle than the insidious, low-level pain he experienced with lupus. "An X-ray plate is very convincing to a doctor and everyone is very supportive," Dr. Nadelson says, "But lupus patients themselves rarely know whether they are tired because of, or for reasons unrelated to, disease." The physician's approach should, first of all, be to assume that if the patient has lupus, fatigue is part of the disease: "It doesn't matter if the doctor is right or wrong; no one in the world can tell." He suggests that the most helpful strategy is to assume that the patients are complaining about something that troubles them, that something is probably going on in their bodies if they say so.

I have heard physicians say that something is strange about the typical lupus patient in particular, something that is very disturbing to them. Many such patients, they say, are hysterical, nagging, highly inquisitive, demanding, anxious, and depressed, and they do not know what this represents, or how to deal with such patients.

Dr. Nadelson says that while he, too, did not know what this typical response represented, when the immune system is not behaving normally, neurological side effects are commonplace. "As a matter of fact," he said, "we are beginning to find that many symptoms we once assumed were separate, almost autonomous, do in fact interact with each other. Lupus probably leads to behavioral changes." Patients with lupus are worried people. They have difficulty managing their everyday affairs, because of the uncertainty and deterioration the disease inflicts on them. If the physician were to imagine struggling through the day weighted down with two forty-pound valises, one in each hand, and, at the same time, being asked to perform normal duties and maintain close loving relationships with family and friends, he or she would get a sense, perhaps, of what lupus patients experience, though only from a psychological point of view. "Add to that the interaction of the nervous system, which is somewhat out of whack because of the disease," Dr. Nadelson said, "and one gets a sense of what it is like to have lupus. Even when patients are seemingly in remission, they still worry about what the future holds and when the next acute attack will come."

How can a psychiatrist help patients with lupus? Dr. Nadelson said: "First of all, lupus is a chameleonlike disease with behavioral manifestations that range all the way from mild depressions to severe psychosis. The issue is further compounded by the fact that patients with lupus are receiving very strong medications, some of which cause behavioral or emotional changes. Steroids, when given in high doses, often cause people to become elated and excited, a condition known as steroid psychosis. When the dose of steroids is rapidly increased or decreased, a normal kind of behavior may return. Lupus itself may produce cerebritis, an irritation of the brain tissue that brings on severe changes in perception. When the patient has a psychosis, whether from drugs or from the irritation caused by the disease, he or she may hallucinate. The degree of the hallucination is usually random, and the hallucinations are usually without structure, depending mostly on the stimuli in the environment. Although steroids can sometimes cause unusual behavioral changes in the patient, they also can be helpful in reducing general inflammation in the body, and therefore decrease behavioral changes caused by brain inflammations."

In Dr. Nadelson's view, patients do generally benefit from supportive psychotherapy, but he thinks that this is not necessarily best delivered by the psychiatrist. Understanding and compassion on the part of the internist can be extremely helpful, he says, in helping the patient through the long process of adaptation to chronic illness. The patient should acknowledge that the disease itself leads to emotional stress. Patients often cannot distinguish the behavioral and emotional difficulties imposed by lupus from problems that existed previously. "Patients very often tend to blame themselves for that which cannot be helped," Dr. Nadelson says. The understanding assurance of the doctor, presented without censure or blame, can greatly help: "This is the dose the doctor should deliver with every medication he or she prescribes."

Dr. Richard Krause, director of the National Institute of Allergy and Infectious Diseases of the National Institutes of Health, says that along with the therapeutic marvels of the past decades, physicians must also add to their black bags a generous portion of "therapon," the Greek word from which therapy is derived, meaning a companion in attendance. Dr. Krause believes that modern medicine may improve the quality of life for patients with chronic diseases, yet it often lacks the capacity to reach out to the patients, to fulfill their needs for guidance and assistance. Dr. Krause does not believe that medicine is devoid of humanity. On the contrary, medicine is as human and as graceful as all of us help to make it.

Shifting lupus patients to psychotherapy, according to Dr. Nadelson, may have a negative effect. The patient may feel that he or she is being discarded because he or she is unacceptable or even "crazy." Sometimes, Dr. Nadelson says, patients may feel they are being sent to someone who can tolerate their craziness because the physician who has been entrusted with the physical disease cannot. He stresses that patients can develop emotional problems in reaction to their illness. Just as we have psychosomatic illness—that is, illness arising from emotional problems—we also have somatopsychic illness; that is, psychological problems that result from a difficult time with physical disease. "Patients with lupus are always wondering about the course of the disease," Dr. Nadelson says. "They often feel as if they are in a dark tunnel with no light at the end. Or they wonder what their eventual situation will be. Troubled with such thoughts, and often without the support of the family or in the midst of an environment that may aggravate the very strain from which they seek relief, the patient turns to the doctor." Dr. Nadelson suggests that a psychiatrist see the patient once or twice, with the idea that their dialogue is going to "help" the physician! The physician may be helped by the knowledge that the psychiatrist is available to counsel him or her in the management of such patients. "The problem doesn't belong only to the patient. Physicians have a real problem in dealing with chronic illness. What they cannot cure makes them frustrated and sometimes even angry at the patient who is not cured."

I thought of a friend of mine, a cardiologist, who is also a lupus patient and is very ill and discouraged. My friend was told by her physician, "Have some equanimity. Most people in this world have to cope with worse." In order to show her how sympathetic he was to her state, he told her about his mother, who was dying of cancer. My friend left the doctor's office feeling disappointed in herself. She was depressed and worried, thinking that she had become a burden not only to herself and family, but also to her physician. The lupus patient is often exposed to veiled criticism for having such a bizarre, little-understood disease. When the physician emphasizes neurosis, that becomes destructive to the whole family, because neurosis implies that the patient has control over the illness. This is not so. Dr. Lucille Carter, a psychiatrist in Boston who works with many lupus patients, has told me that patients in such a situation are forced to make themselves live as normal people, even though lupus patients have less strength and healthy energy.

Dr. Malcolm P. Rogers, Assistant Professor of Psychiatry at Harvard University Medical School, and Assistant Director of Psychiatry, Brigham and Women's Hospital, ascribes the confusion over whether neurotics fall prey to lupus, or lupus creates neurotics, to a combination of factors: "the frequent lag time in diagnosis, the intense emotions triggered by the disease, and the potential for direct involvement of the brain through inflammation."

As has been discussed earlier, the fact that lupus involves symptoms and signs in many different parts of the body, frequently at different times, makes it difficult to diagnose. Many of its symptoms, such as fatigue and aches and pains, are not specific. Some patients will have been ill for a prolonged period of time, during which not much physically wrong with them will have been found. Suspicions about whether their illness might be psychosomatic may well have arisen, and, as a matter of fact, need to be considered as part of the differential diagnosis when physical symptoms seem inconsistent. Sensitive exploration of such a possibility is usually accepted by patients. However, feelings of anger, mistrust, and self-doubt may develop during this early phase of diagnostic confusion and can have residual effects on later encounters with doctors. Occasionally, for these reasons, lupus patients may be perceived as neurotic by doctors.

A psychiatrist would approach this question by trying to determine the lupus patient's usual mental state and personality and then reconstructing when and how it changed. This baseline personality becomes the normal standard against which change is measured. When was he or she last "himself" or "herself" and how is he or she different? In the case of lupus, it is the doctor who needs to listen empathetically to the major losses this illness has created. He or she should decide whether the patient's reactions are neurotic or appropriate, given the magnitude of the recent adjustment. Probably the most important question is whether the behavior and emotional states are adaptive for successful functioning in relationships with friends and family, for work, and for optimal care within the medical community. In essence, the doctor must try to make a very complicated judgment about whether the level of fear—or depression, or anger, or whatever emotional reaction—is part of a constructive coping process, or rather suggests that the patient is overwhelmed. The perspective of the family is invaluable in this assessment. Depending on the outcome of this evaluation, the patient's primary doctor may raise the possibility of psychiatric care to help the patient regain his or her emotional equilibrium. The suggestion of psychiatric care should not be misperceived as minimizing the difficulties of the disease itself, or as an implication that the patient is "crazy" or weak. The illness requires working through many readjustments, and sometimes the intervention of a skilled mental-health professional knowledgeable about the disease can be extremely beneficial.

As mentioned earlier, other factors of lupus can affect the patient's mental state. One factor is the inflammation in the brain (lupus cerebritis); the other is the effect on mood and memory caused by the use of prednisone (or other corticosteroids). When intellectual capacities such as memory or attention span become impaired (with or without other emotional changes), a diagnosis of lupus cerebritis is more likely. Unfortunately, documenting the diagnosis of lupus cerebritis is frequently very difficult. For obvious reasons, brain biopsies are not performed for this purpose, and the neurological diagnostic procedures generally used—lumbar puncture, CAT scan, EEG—are not always sensitive enough to detect lupus cerebritis when it is present. Special psychological tests for memory and attention can be helpful in diagnosis, but a still more sensitive neurophysiological test is needed. New brain imaging techniques may offer such a possibility in the future. "All in all," Dr. Rogers says, "sorting out what mental processes may be reaction to disease as opposed to manifestations of the disease itself, and attempting to gauge their adaptiveness, is a complicated matter for both patient and physician."

Is a more general therapy necessary for lupus patients? Dr. Carter suggests that we look again at some of the problems lupus patients must face. First, they must deal with the shock of learning they have a complicated, chronic illness that may alter, sometimes dramatically, all their plans and dreams for their lives. Some of the questions such patients may face and with which they may have to struggle are: How will this illness disturb normal life? How will you react to the changes? How will your family react? Your husband or wife, children, relatives? What differences will there be in your friendships (e.g., can you participate in sports and entertaining)? Will you be thought of as ill? How will you handle the drain and stress? How will those close to you stand the vagaries of the disease?

If you are working, what difference will your illness make in your drive for success? Is a second income needed?

How will you handle the blows to self-esteem? How will you keep your spirits up? How will you value yourself now? How will you think of yourself as a marriage partner, including dealing with sexual needs? How will the illness affect mothering? And housekeeping?

"Surely," Dr. Carter emphasizes, "one can see the need for support of some type. Therapy can help. The lupus patient may be fortunate to have a physician who knows how to ease things and work toward patient participation in treatment. However, several other types of support are available, because physicians can't do it all. A psychiatrist trained in chronic disease may be the wisest choice in some circumstances," she says, and points out that other helpful insights are offered by especially trained nurses, psychologists, and social workers. Workshops and self-help groups may also be beneficial.

Understanding the problems of chronic disease in a loved one can be difficult. As Dr. Nadelson and Dr. Rogers explain, all these problems are further complicated by reaction to medication. Dr. Carter feels that patients need to take an active part in their treatment. "All this is to help patients reduce their burden," she says, "so they should reach out for assistance. They should ask for it."

Many patients write: "I have lupus and have been seeing my doctor for over a year now. I don't think that I am making enough progress and wonder whether someone else might be able to do more for me. But I worry that my doctor will be upset if I seek another opinion. What should I do?"

Dr. Rogers says a second opinion may be a good idea. As suggested earlier, if a patient is in doubt about whether to follow a particular treatment, he or she has every right to review it with another physician. "Don't hide such a decision from your doctor," he says. "In fact, as a common courtesy, you should let your doctor know whom you are planning to see and why. The outside consultant will generally want to see a summary of your medical record anyway. Your own doctor should welcome such outside consultation. Confirmation of his or her treatment plan by another physician can only strengthen it and help you to comply with the treatment. On the other hand, if a well-qualified consultant recommends a different course of action, your doctor may welcome that as valuable input. He or she may disagree, and ultimately the patient will have to judge which person or recommendation is the more compelling. In some situations, your doctor may feel that it should not be in your best interest to seek another opinion. And he or she may be right. The key to it is that your physician should always be acting in your best interest, not his or hers. If your physician's ego seems wounded, if he or she is offended or angered by your decisison, that is your physician's problem and not yours."*

At another meeting with Dr. Nadelson, he showed me a videotape he made of his session with a lupus patient in the psychiatric ward of the hospital. His approach was gentle, philosophical. He allowed the patient to reminisce as long as she wanted, giving her the feeling that he would gladly listen even if she rambled or philosophized a little. The patient talked for a few moments about her childhood,

* Malcolm Rogers, M.D., "Should You Seek a Second Medical Opinion?" *Lupus News*, Winter 1984.

describing her lack of concentration in school, her forgetfulness, and the fatigue she had experienced most of her life. The patient spoke of her changes in mood, of anxiety and depression. Then she described how strict her mother had been with her, how she never believed that she was really ill, how she herself wondered if she was sick or simply lazy. She was conscious always of a feeling of guilt. Yet she did not really know what she might have done wrong. The patient went on describing how unfair and difficult her life had been and how angry and resentful she felt about it. "I needed my mother's understanding," the patient said, "but above all I needed her love."

The woman remained quiet for a moment, and then her face unexpectedly lit up with a smile.

"You are smiling for the first time," Dr. Nadelson said. "What are you thinking of?"

"My children," the woman said.

"What about your children?" he asked.

The woman's smile broadened. "I am happy that I can still love my children in my own way," she answered.

The woman's words contained a good deal of feeling. I wondered whether her love for her children would give her the emotional strength to overcome the hardships of this illness. Patients have told me that they have developed self-hatred because of what the disease does to their body and soul. They say that such hatred projects itself into every part of their lives, including their relationships with the people they love. But this was not one of the woman's problems.

I asked Dr. Malcolm Rogers how important is the will to recover in a patient. And if it is lost, what can be done to recover it? Dr. Rogers answered that a patient's will to recover is very important. He wrote the following to be included in this chapter:

"Although some philosophical treatises have doubted the very existence of 'will' in human action, few experienced clinicians can fail to be impressed with its importance in health and illness. A similar state of disease in two different patients (as far as it can be measured objectively) may lead to total disability in one or to a mild annoyance in another. Patients also exercise considerable will in their choice of medical help, and in their (often underestimated) capacity to elicit maximum care, or avoidance, as the case may be. In addition, regardless of the treatment prescribed, the patient has the choice to follow it or not, or to assume an active or passive role with the physician in the pursuit of health. Patients may be victims of a disease, but not helpless victims.

"The sudden onset of a disease such as lupus frequently does lead to a feeling of helplessness, however. One of the hardest things about this disease, which begins so mysteriously within one's body, is that it tends to undermine a person's sense of inner control. People are used to controlling their own bodies. Suddenly, fatigue, aches and pains, and skin rashes begin and do not vanish after the expected interval. No matter what the patient does, these symptoms linger in unfamiliar and inexplicable ways. This is, in fact, how people begin to recognize that they may have a disease. Sometimes, however, before the disease is clearly identified, patients may encounter doubt and disbelief in others about the existence of these symptoms. Sometimes they may encounter such reactions in their doctors. Sometimes, even worse, they may begin to doubt themselves and their own perceptions. Not surprisingly, therefore, some patients lose their will, at least temporarily. Not only have they been betrayed by their own bodies, but also their experience has been invalidated. For most patients, fortunately, this feeling of helplessness will be relatively brief. Time, understanding, support, and a treatment plan will reverse it. Gradually, patients begin to identify what is within their control and what is beyond it, and focus their energy on that which they can control.

"Sometimes the feeling of helplessness and loss of will persist. Their persistence may signal the existence of a serious clinical depression, in which case it will be accompanied by feelings of sadness, hopelessness, loss of concentration, loss of interest and pleasure, and a disturbance of sleep and appetite. Suicidal thoughts may occur. Patients caught in the web of this kind of depression need prompt attention from a psychiatrist. Treatment generally consists of specific antidepressant medication and psychotherapy. The psychiatrist must also consider the possibility that lupus involving the brain itself might be responsible for such a mental change.

"In the more typical situations, however, a feeling of helplessness will be transient. Expressions of this feeling tend to mobilize caring and support in others, at least for a while. Patients do need help both from the physical demands and from the responsibilities of everyday life. Their energy needs to be diverted temporarily into coping with the disease. Getting over the initial shock, grieving for the loss of health and the other capacities undercut by this illness takes time. Patients will call upon inner strengths that have helped them through previous crises. They will gradually learn to accept the reality of the illness and learn more about lupus. They will begin to develop a treatment plan, together with their doctor, and a personal strategy for dealing with their illness on a day-to-day or week-to-week basis. Patients cannot by an act of will make their illness disappear, but they can, by an act of will, refuse to let it destroy their spirit.

"Most patients, including the lupus patient, expect to receive medical care that is not only technologically advanced, but also sensitive to their human needs. They want their physicians to respond in a personal, sensitive fashion and show more understanding of how a disease can affect a human life. Many patients feel that without understanding this, the physicians cannot properly treat the patient. In theory, most doctors vigorously espouse the importance of humanism in medicine. In practice the task is, of course, much harder. It is worth considering some of the pressures that make it so."

"At the heart of the problem of 'humanism in medicine' is the growth of specialization and subspecialization," Dr. Rogers says. The therapeutic advances in medicine in the past fifty years have been dramatic. No one doctor can master all the diagnostic and therapeutic options currently available, ranging from CAT scans to the latest in microsurgery or chemotherapy. The technological benefits are accompanied, inevitably, by a greater fragmentation of care. In his book entitled *The Youngest Science: Notes of a Medicine-Watcher*, Lewis Thomas traces the recent history of the radical transformation of medicine in his own career and even in his own experience as a patient. After describing his hospitalization for gastrointestinal bleeding, Dr. Thomas writes that the incident had been his first personal experience with the kind of illness requiring hospital technology. Thinking back, he considered that his treatment had been perfectly satisfactory, but nevertheless he felt that for much of his hospital stay he had been treated more like an object on an assembly line than a person: "While it was going on I felt less like a human in trouble and more like a scientific problem to be solved as quickly as possible. What made it work, and kept such notions as 'depersonalization' and 'dehumanization' from even popping into my mind, was the absolute confidence and skill of the people who had hold of me."

For patients with lupus, the trend toward increasing specialization in medicine has had both its pluses and its minuses, Dr. Rogers says. On the plus side, doctors trained in rheumatology and immunology have made important research advances and developed special expertise in dealing with lupus. On the minus side, many patients feel that the specialists they had seen early on, often before the diagnosis was made, examined them in a fragmented, noncommital fashion. Many did not look beyond the organ system of their own specialty. They often did not feel responsible to the patient as a whole. In more recent years, the development of primary-care practice in internal medicine has evolved, in part, to counter such fragmentation in medical practice.

Dr. Rogers stresses that other pressures, in the 1980s, may oppose the style of practice that is characterized by a genuine caring for the patient. Economic and bureaucratic pressures are having an increasing impact. Potential financial incentives tend to reward technical procedures and to discourage less well-defined time simply spent talking with the patient. Dr. Rogers quotes from a recent article in the *New England Journal of Medicine*, which presents a facetious complaint of a health-care bureaucrat against a physician who fails to conform to these new demands ("The Unfortunate Case of Dr. Z: How to Succeed in Medical Practice in 1984," March 15, 1984): "Dr. Z's rebellious obstinacy first came to our attention in the early 1970s. . . . From the very outset, he failed to submit diagnoses that matched the computer disease and procedure codes. What was more, he refused to accept the guiding principles of the new medicine," that any illness could be completely defined by a diagnosis for which there was a corresponding treatment.

The article continues to document many of Dr. Z's "crimes," which include his claims that patients came to see him for a number of reasons other than for the diagnosis of a specific ailment: to establish themselves with a regular physician; for regular physical checkups; to allay their fears of disease; for genetic counseling; for advice on overseas travel; to hear his opinion on surgery or new medications; or even simply to have someone to talk to about their troubles. Dr. Z even made the "outrageous" assertion that a single disease might be just one of many, differing in severity from person to person, with emotional and psychological components. Dr. Z concluded, complains the bureaucrat, that each person's illness was unique, and therefore "the patients' feelings, their reactions to their disease, count."

Dr. Rogers's answer to Dr. Z's suggestion, of course, is that we have no code or criteria for what he calls "personal care."

Dr. Rogers explains that the capacity to resist these pressures lies both in the character of physicians and in the nature of the training they receive. Medical students can and should be selected not only for their academic abilities but for their interpersonal skills as well. Their teachers and the hospitals where they train should emphasize that medicine is an ethical, not a commercial enterprise. They will learn in large measure by imitating their teachers or models. And if the marketplace is allowed to operate, patients themselves will insist on an emphasis on access and personal care. Ultimately, patients will insist that their doctors understand them as people.

The era of specialization is here to stay, Dr. Rogers says, and can offer much to the patient as long as it is well enough integrated. To some degree, the field of consultation-liaison psychiatry has developed to facilitate the integration between technological and psychological medicine. As Dr. Z. J. Lipowski, a well-known spokesman for this field, has pointed out, the roots of this discipline date back at least to the work of Benjamin Rush (1745–1813), commonly considered to be the founder of American psychiatry, who spoke in his day of the reciprocal influence of the body and mind as a "single and indivisible being, for so intimately united are his soul and body that one cannot be moved, without the other." Liaison psychiatry has flourished largely since World War II, reintegrating psychiatry and medicine, Dr. Rogers says. He points out that Lipowski defines liaison psychiatry as "that subdivision of clinical psychiatry which involves consultation to and collaboration with nonpsychiatric physicians in all types of medical settings, but especially in general hospitals. It is primarily concerned with problems of diagnosis, management, study, and prevention of psychiatric morbidity in the physically ill and those who manifest their psychological distress in the form of somatic complaints."*

Dr. Rogers stresses that the practical benefit for many patients

* Z. S. Lipowski, *American Journal of Psychiatry*, 138, 1981.

with lupus is that psychiatric help, if needed, should be provided by someone who knows the essential medical realities of their disease, and is used to working in close collaboration with their medical physicians.

Liaison psychiatry has also focused attention on the doctor-patient relationship: what stresses it and what strengthens it. Doctors can benefit by reflecting on their own emotional responses to patients and illness. Dr. Thomas's account of his own illness certainly emphasizes the importance of the patient's perception of the doctor. The course of any illness is thoroughly intertwined with a multitude of psychological and social issues, which, as Dr. Z points out, have major effects on the outcome. Patients will not feel understood by their doctors unless they can communicate their experience of the illness, and such understanding is a crucial component of caring for the patient.

9

Nursing:
A Vital Role in Lupus Care

Nurses play an important role in helping the lupus patient cope with the disease. They also play a role as a liaison between the physician, the scientist, the patient, and the family. I asked Dr. Tamara Bethel, R.N., Ph.D., to address some of these issues in this chapter. Dr. Bethel is on the faculty of Newton-Wellesley Hospital School of Nursing; she is trained in psychiatric nursing and has a good insight into the plight of the lupus patient.

Dr. Bethel is directly responsible for Chronicare '84, a program and curriculum for community-based nurses on the care of patients with chronic diseases (see Chapter 17).

The Newton-Wellesley Hospital is a major teaching institution associated with Tufts University Medical School and the New England Medical Center.

Dr. Bethel has the following comments: "Nurses traditionally find themselves in the position of being the persons who are with patients in hospitals for the greatest cumulative amount of time. They have the unique advantage of seeing patients in all phases of their illnesses, exhibiting all the symptoms that they will exhibit, behaving in all the ways that they will behave, and, in general, being all the personalities that they can and will be. The nurse will be called upon to respond to all the pain and discomfort, confusion and fright, anger and anxiety that the patient will demonstrate. In addition, nurses also have the great opportunity to share in the good times, the remissions of illness, or the elation of finding a treatment that brings relief from suffering or pain. Often, it is the nurse who can be instrumental in keeping that realistic hope for tomorrow alive in the patient. For these and for many other reasons that will be addressed in this chapter, we see a valuable opportunity for nurses to be an integral part of the medical team that treats persons with such chronic diseases as lupus.

"Lupus may be a very insidious disease, and some special nursing problems may occur in the care of certain patients. The person with the disease may go undiagnosed for many years. Indeed, the vague symptoms of extreme fatigue, generalized weakness, anorexia, and weight loss may cause the patient to spend many months and more dollars going from doctor to doctor, hospital to hospital, clinic to clinic, in search of a diagnosis that is treatable. If fever, rash, and/or joint involvement are present in the constellation of symptoms, the picture may become even more complicated instead of more concrete. The patient may become even more exhausted in the quest for some medical help and may soon begin to doubt herself and the validity of her complaints. "Do you think I'm going crazy?" is a common remark made in an offhanded way to a trusted nurse who has taken the time to listen.

"To feel as if one is losing control is, in itself, an extremely frightening sensation. It is no more frightening if the control in question is of a physical nature than if it is of an emotional nature, as comments such as those above indicate. Mrs. C. was a patient in the local community hospital. She had been involved for several weeks in searching for a diagnosis and treatment that would bring her relief from her many physical symptoms, including joint pain, a transient rash, nausea, extreme fatigue, and anxiety about her symptoms. The nurses caring for her were becoming increasingly frustrated by Mrs. C.'s behavior, which included keeping voluminous notes in journals of all her symptoms as well as her interactions with the staff. In addition, she spent a great deal of time on the telephone calling physician after physician, often in the late-night hours, often at their homes, and always to the utter chagrin of the staff on the floor, who subsequently incurred the irritation of the physician for 'not controlling that woman's access to the telephone.' As Mrs. C.'s attempts to control what was happening to her increased, it became more and more difficult for the staff to respond to her in ways that were appropriate to her needs. Instead, a great deal of energy was expended in reacting to her seemingly unreasonable attempts to obtain some relief from her feelings of having no control over what was happening to her. She was a patient on a busy medical teaching unit in the hospital; she was being poked and prodded, tested and questioned continuously by a never-ending stream of well-meaning interns, residents, students, physicians, nurses, and consultants; and she was still feeling that no one knew exactly what was wrong with her or whether, indeed, there was anything wrong with her that wasn't 'all in her head.' It was at this point, several weeks into her hospitalization, that one of the staff nurses who worked evenings began some meaningful interactions and interventions with Mrs. C. This nurse, Peg, accurately assessed Mrs. C.'s behavior as that of someone who was frightened, not angry and demanding as everyone else had construed her behavior. Peg took the time to sit with Mrs. C. and talk about her feelings. Peg helped her to see that her behavior and her actions were not getting her the result that she intended, but were in fact making her feel worse as people were avoiding her for fear of being written up in Mrs. C.'s journals. In talking with this nurse later, it was clear that she had been able to make a difference both in the attitudes of Mrs. C. toward what was happening to her and in the attitudes of some of the other persons who had come in contact with this patient. While the fact of the matter was that this nurse tried an approach of sitting and listening, of taking time out from a busy schedule and a heavy patient load to do what she did, she did it of necessity. Mrs. C., in her feelings of losing control, was controlling the behavior of everyone on the unit and was not aware of it. Many persons were not receiving what they needed because of the fruitless energies that were being misdirected into reacting to Mrs. C.'s chaotic attempts to get help. As she tried desperately to find some relief from her feelings of being frightened and isolated, she structured situations that caused more confusion and more avoidance behavior. She therefore contributed to further isolation and more confusing, scary situations. Although Peg's motives may not have been the purest (she needed to be able to spend more time with her other patients), she did exactly what was needed when she spent more positive time with Mrs. C. In responding to Mrs. C.'s need to regain control, Peg, in fact, gained more control over her work as well. She ended up spending the same amount of time with Mrs. C., and they both benefited from it, because the time became more goal-directed toward the need that Mrs. C. had to feel less frightened, more informed of the agenda for her care, and more in charge of her own destiny.

"As a result of these interventions, Peg was also able to help Mrs. C. with another problem she was experiencing, a very negative concept of herself. Two other patients, Connie and Lucy, had a similar problem with feeling different because they were living with a chronic disease such as lupus. Connie was an eighteen-year-old black woman who was attending school in the Boston area. She had left her home in the Southwest to attend Wellesley College as a freshman. Prior to her diagnosis of lupus, Connie had exhibited symptoms of arthralgias, rashes on her forearms, back, trunk and legs, and low grade fevers for about four to six months. While she never felt truly ill, she was very concerned that she never felt quite well and consequently was not able to participate in activities that her classmates were involved in. In addition, she became worried when she developed oral ulcers. When her boyfriend expressed a wish to terminate their relationship, she became even more isolated and withdrawn than she had previously been. She was accompanied to the emergency unit of the local hospital by a dorm advisor because she seemed depressed and sick and was talking about not having any friends and being a mess.

"Connie was, indeed, very ill at the time, and in addition to the lupus flare she was experiencing, she had some serious problems with depression. Connie had not yet had a diagnosis made of lupus, so she was totally unable to understand the symptoms she was having. She was feeling helpless, hopeless, abandoned by her boyfriend, homesick, and ostracized because of what she perceived as symptoms of some horrible, dirty disease. She saw herself as being disfigured by the ulcers in her mouth and the discolorations caused by the rashes on her face and body. Within a short time, a positive diagnosis of lupus was established, and appropriate medical treatment was initiated. It was left to others to deal with this pathetic young woman and her low self-esteem. Fortunately, Connie was receptive to interactions from the student nurses who cared for her. They were her age; some of them were also away from home for the first time and had some similar experiences to share with her. It became an important time for Connie to begin to relate to other people in a positive, open manner. She could share some of her experiences as a newcomer to the Boston area, and the student nurses could share with Connie some of the things they were learning about lupus. Connie's feelings of helplessness and hopelessness were soon replaced by feelings of friendship and warmth toward these people who were able to respond to her with such positivity. They treated Connie almost as if she were one of their classmates, and invited her and her physician to give a talk to the class about lupus. They told her that there were cosmetologists who specialized in skin disorders and were able to help her select appropriate cosmetics to make her rash less noticeable. In addition, because Connie had been seen by so many different consultants in the hospital, it became difficult for Connie to keep track of all the various approaches and suggestions that were given her. The student nurses initiated a system for Connie that helped her sort out some of the information she was getting and to use it appropriately. When the students were having classes in assertiveness training, they practiced the lessons with Connie. As a result, Connie herself became much more assertive and was able to take some control of her treatment and her interactions with the various clinicians treating her. As Connie learned more about her illness, she became better able to manage some of her symptoms. She was also able to adjust her schedule to accommodate adequate rest and was able to feel better, look better, and act better. She became a more interesting and vital person, began to attract more friends, and consequently, felt less isolated and depressed.

"Lucy presented a much different picture than either of the two patients described previously. Lucy was thirteen years old when the nurses on her unit first saw her. She had been diagnosed as having lupus when she was nine years old and now, at thirteen, was having her fifth hospital admission for pulse therapy (the administration of high doses of steroids intravenously for three to five days). In about four and a half years with the disease, Lucy had never truly been in remission. She had well-documented SLE with mild to moderate renal disease, fevers, low levels of white blood cells, moderate hemolytic anemia, arthralgias, arthritis, and rashes. When admitted this fifth time, she had high fevers and a cough, but her only joint pain was in her elbow, and she seemed proud of the fact that she got the sore elbow after throwing snowballs at some of the other kids in the neighborhood who were laughing at her and making fun of her. Except for this one spark of emotion that she displayed when talking about standing up for herself, she was generally seen as too quiet and appeared depressed.

"Lucy looked quite Cushingoid (i.e., had a moonface) due to the steroids that she had been taking. She was able to talk about her problems with the other children in the group at school making fun of her appearance. In addition, she needed some special attention in school, as she was prone to nosebleeds, occasional diarrhea, and frequent absences due to upper respiratory or urinary tract infections. In spite of all this, she managed to maintain an A average. Because she had been diagnosed for so long and because she was so bright, Lucy presented special problems. Her age and the serious nature of her involvement made symptomatic treatment difficult. Steroids were of some help, but pulse therapy did not have a profound enough effect to warrant continued use. In addition, dosages of steroids every other day did not relieve her tiredness, and she began to have intermittent headaches, chest pain, and other vague symptoms indicating this was not the correct approach to treatment either. Lucy was generally compliant with her prescribed treatment but had some difficulty with 'feeling and being different.' She was 'sick of having to make up schoolwork.' She wanted to be like the other kids but saw this as impossible as she had to maintain a special diet, stay out of sunlight, limit the exposure she had to fluorescent lights, and take the other precautions that were specific to her treatment. She also saw herself as fat, as some of the other kids had been calling her, and at that very important age of thirteen and a half, it is important to be like one's friends in almost every way. Lucy saw herself as nothing like any of her friends: they did not have special diets, or too many extra pounds or nosebleeds. They had plenty of energy and interests, could go to the beach and sunbathe—all things that were definitely not options for Lucy. The only thing that she had going for her was her A average, as far as she was concerned.

"Lucy was ably and competently treated by some of the best scientists, physicians, and clinicians in a major medical center. They were all acutely aware of this young girl's physical symptoms and the treatments that would give her the best chance of remission. Unfortunately, not one of these staff members was available during visiting hours in the hospital. Not one of them was aware of the fact that although Lucy's parents and grandparents were attentive and regular visitors, Lucy did not have any visitors her own age for the entire time that she was hospitalized, for any of her six hospitalizations in the four years she was known to the medical center. Not only that, but Lucy did not socialize with any of the other adolescents that were in the hospital at the same time she was. Once again, the nursing staff was responsible for picking up this lack of socialization on Lucy's part. It was noted that another patient on the floor at the time was from Lucy's school. When approached about this, Lucy told the nurse that she did not know any of the kids from school because they were all afraid to be with her because she was always sick. When the nurse approached the other patient, Susan, and asked if she knew Lucy, Susan replied that she did know her because they were in the same class, but that she found it hard to talk to her because she was 'funny' acting. Some careful manipulations on the part of the nurse brought Lucy and Susan together a few times, and with the support of the nursing staff, the two girls found things in common to talk about. Lucy was able to help Susan with some of her schoolwork, and Susan was able to tell Lucy about some of the other kids in the school who "weren't so bad." Lucy and Susan are not best friends today, but that one observation on the part of the nursing staff was instrumental in helping Lucy to see herself and some of her abilities in a more realistic light and to realize that maybe she was different, but even so, she had something to offer to others. The nurses' knowledge of child growth and development as well as the ability to look at the total picture of the patient was critical in helping a youngster in ways that go beyond the best treatment by the best scientists, physicians, and clinicians.

"Lucy experienced an unfortunate incident while she was being treated in this famous medical center. As is the style of such large teaching centers, the physicians, consultants, interns, and residents on the service, as well as the medical students, conducted rounds at the bedside of each patient regularly. After examining the patient and asking each other questions about their findings, they discuss the case, sometimes right at the bedside or right outside the door. They often seem to forget that the patient is listening to what they are saying. Although the patient may be very articulate and have a good and accurate knowledge and understanding of his or her disease and symptoms, he or she may hear information that may not be related to the patient or may be in an inappropriate context. In Lucy's case, she heard the group discussing her poor prognosis because of the age of onset of her disease and the severity of symptoms she had at various times. As a result, Lucy became very depressed and acted out for a period by being noncompliant with treatment and negativistic about her one accomplishment—her schoolwork—and in general becoming a nasty young lady for a few days. While no one could quite understand what had happened to cause this turnaround in her usual behavior, everyone knew that something had caused it, and finally Lucy herself let the staff in on the problem. During one of the usual great hubbubs of teaching rounds, Lucy very nastily asked the doctors why they were bothering with her if she had such a poor prognosis. The group was quite surprised to hear her speaking of this, and were forced to look at their own communications! It is a lesson that none in that team will soon forget.

"The three patients described above are but a few that have benefited from some meaningful interventions by primary caretakers who were nurses. All of the patients had exquisite and competent care and treatment by any number of highly skilled scientists and physicians—dermatologists, nephrologists, rheumatologists, pediatricians, general physicians, hematologists, and other lupus specialists. In each of the cases described, however, there seemed to be a missing link. While all the experts addressed each other and the textbook problems of lupus, no one seemed intent on having conversations with the actual patient. Someone needed to be responsible for pulling all the various pieces of information together for and with the patient and for helping the patient integrate this information into the total scheme of his or her life. In at least the three cases cited, it was the nurse who was in the best position to do this. The nurse has the background and scientific base of information to assist the patient to integrate the findings of the examinations. He or she is able to look at the patient with a caring, persistent, trusting approach and communicate with the humanistic and spiritual touch that is the missing link between the highly scientific and highly technical data generated by today's medical investigators. Because nurses are one of the few constant factors in the patient's hospital experience, they are able to identify behaviors the patient may demonstrate which indicate that he or she is fearful, has questions, is concerned about things other than the results of lab tests, does not understand what is happening or is being said to him or her. Nurses can help the patient to learn how and what to communicate to other persons involved in his or her care. They can be the one constant resource for assisting patients in finding the answers to questions related to health, illness, treatment, or even managing social matters and financial affairs. The contact with the nurse does not necessarily have to end with discharge from the hospital. There are nurses in virtually every setting who can be used by patients in the many ways cited above. For these important reasons, nurses are increasingly seeing themselves as the important liaison between the physician, the scientist, the patient and his or her family, and the other members of the health-care team."

10

The Latest Addition
to the Health Care Team:
The Dentist

A lupus patient wrote: "I am in constant pain. Every bone in my body feels on fire, and so does my jaw. Upon examination the dentist could not find anything wrong. He gave me a painkiller and promised the pain would go away. The family doctor told me that my facial pain was caused by nerves. He increased the Valium and told me to stop looking in the mirror. Recently I went to see a dental surgeon. He emphasized the importance of a proper diagnosis of symptoms such as mine because of a number of different medical and dental conditions that could cause further complications. He advised me to check in the mirror for possible facial changes."

I thought this patient's story was an isolated case. However, since then I have spoken to several other patients who complained of changes in the position of their mouths and of acute pain in their jaws. Flannery O'Connor, who suffered from lupus, described in one of her books the changes in the position of her mouth. From her description, it appears that her lupus affected her bones, both her jaw and her hips.

Lupus patients have many oral and dental difficulties that add to the confusing picture of the disease. They complain of fungal infections in their mouths, changes in the texture of their saliva, and difficulties tolerating partial dentures in their mouths because of inflammation and bleeding gums. Others are allergic to local anesthetics and to some antibiotics prescribed by dentists unaware of the potential adverse reactions experienced by some of these patients.

I have been with the same dentist for more than thirty years, and we still remember how ignorant we were about lupus and the oral complications caused by the disease. I had bleeding gums, ulcerations on the insides of my cheeks, small pockets of infection deep inside the gums, and cavities close to the gum line. I've heard patients calling themselves "dental cripples," and I almost became one.

When I spoke to the Lupus Society of Quebec some months ago, I learned that Dr. Martin T. Tyler had presented an outstanding lecture on this subject. After the meeting, I called Dr. Tyler at his home, and he agreed to meet with me the following morning.

Dr. Tyler is with the Montreal General Hospital Dental Clinic (Oral Diagnosis) and is an assistant professor and chairman of oral diagnosis and dental radiology at McGill University in Montreal. He has a deep interest in the welfare of the lupus patient. I told Dr. Tyler that I understood from some of my friends at the meeting that he works in an area of dentistry with special competence relating to patients with oral problems like those experienced by the lupus patient.

"I have additional training in oral diagnosis and oral medicine that focuses on diagnosis and treatment of oral disease, but changes have occurred in the dental-school curriculum that have moved the dentist from the mechanical to the biomedical approach of total patient care," Dr. Tyler reported. "Today's dentist should be prepared to assume the responsibility for the care of special patients like the lupus patient. I cannot say with honesty that all physicians and dentists are as aware of or as experienced with the lupus patient as we would like, but, as I mentioned, changes in the curriculum and more importantly, the push for more involvement in continuing education can be expected to correct this deficiency. The professional dental organizations have realized that if they do not assume the responsibility of encouraging continuing education, outside governmental bodies will. Every professional wants autonomy, and I think the dental organizations and the individual dentists are shouldering their responsibilities."

Lupus patients can help promote awareness among the dental community by supporting continuing education in two areas: urging the dental societies to include pertinent programs in the continuing education curriculum, and encouraging active involvement by dentists in both the educational and organizational pursuits of the local and national lupus societies. Dr. Tyler emphasized that many of his colleagues would volunteer in the educational and organizational activities if approached. The individual not only serves the patients and lupus organizations, but involvement also increases his or her awareness and knowledge. This increased involvement can become contagious to colleagues.

Dr. Tyler believes that organizational involvement with patient education is absolutely necessary to help the patient accept and manage the disease, but a team approach of doctor and patient also needs to be emphasized. "The role of patient education, whether it pertains to the control of gum disease or dental caries, is now a primary function of the family dentist. The lupus patient has special needs that must be pointed out and monitored with regularity."

What specific needs are unique to the lupus patient?

"All patients need to master basic techniques of home care," Dr. Tyler said, since most patients have some level of chronic gum infection. "Infection in the lupus patient may be more severe, especially in those taking systemic corticosteroids such as prednisone. Early diagnosis and treatment of incipient fungal infections that are common to many systemically weakened patients is a routine procedure for the knowledgeable dentist. A small percentage of patients have lupus anticoagulant in their blood, which may cause bleeding. Routine dental tests available to any knowledgeable doctor can eliminate this danger. Of major significance is the fact that many lupus patients don't produce enough saliva and may have a dry mouth. The decrease in output of saliva can result in rampant caries of teeth, and preventive measures must be taken. The preventive procedures consist mainly of special, rather inexpensive appliances that are custom-made for the topical application of fluoride to the teeth. This technique, known to all family dentists, will dramatically reduce or prevent tooth decay in the patient with a dry mouth" (xerostomia).

Dr. Tyler stressed that the dentist may be the first one of the health team to help diagnose disorders, since the average patient sees his or her dentist more frequently than his or her physician.

Disorders such as dry mouth and dry eyes and a medical history of involvement of the joints will alert astute dentists to order routine laboratory studies and to consult with and refer the patient to the appropriate physician for definitive diagnosis and treatment. "A few patients have joint diseases that accompany lupus," Dr. Tyler said. "This is usually very benign and will resolve. However, dentists are familiar with jaw-joint (temporomandibular joint) disorders. With conservative, nonsurgical procedures, discomfort can usually be alleviated."

Another area in dentistry needs to be emphasized. "One important fact is that the dental patient is under additional stress. It is stressful to go to the dentist, even for routine care. The fear of the possibility of discomfort is stressful. Apprehensive patients must receive sympathetic understanding, and the lupus patient especially must be treated with T.L.C. to avoid possible exacerbation of systemic problems. Medications are also an important consideration. Not only may the dentist be stripped of his or her normal tools—antibiotics to control infection, sedatives to control stress, and anodynes to control discomfort—but the patient is many times on multiple medications. These medications must be considered before prescribing others to avoid possible ill effects. Again, these are problems that a dentist on the alert can manage."

In the future, perhaps the Lupus Foundation of America will bring the dental problems of the lupus patient to the attention of health-insurance companies. They should recognize that oral and dental problems can be part of the disease.

PART III

LIVING WITH LUPUS

11

A Personal Account
of Living with Lupus

As I describe later in this chapter, I must have had a genetic predisposition to lupus all my life. However, I was not diagnosed with lupus until after my last child was born in 1953.

The diagnosis was made after three years of intensive searching by Dr. George W. Torn, who, as chief of medicine, was the catalyst who mobilized the brainpower and resources of Harvard's Peter Bent Brigham Hospital (now Brigham and Women's Hospital) toward the relief of my suffering.

After my kidneys collapsed when my disease was in full bloom, there were many nights when I could not sleep, and I asked myself: What is my greatest fear? The answer, invariably, was: How would my children live if I were to die? How could I leave them alone? And what could I do to help them? In talking to other patients, I found that every person has a reason for wanting to stay alive, and the reasons are not the same for each. For me, it was my children's need to have a mother. Others have a passion for work, or love for nature, or for music. One lupus patient I know clings to life because he likes to eat and has a passion for dry martinis!

During those days of fears and apprehensions, I had frightening nightmares. When I woke up in the darkness, I was aware of unclear images that frightened me into a cold sweat. I stared into the darkness until the fading grays killed all images in the dimness of the dream.

143

Then the room lightened, reflecting the paleness of the morning sky, and I could feel a change to reality. Some nights I sat up, afraid to lie down again, and on other nights I walked into the garden, waiting for the burst of light on the horizon, and the realization that I was alive. On such nights I could feel myself chilling, then everything gave way to tears. When I returned to bed, my husband was always asleep. He slept, unaware of my fears and the panic that had settled in my heart. As my body warmed up, I fell into a dreamless sleep in which everything became obliterated by repose. I do not believe that nightmares express a secret wish for death. My nightmares were caused by feelings of fatigue and helplessness and the fear of becoming dependent on others like a child.

Despite the passage of time, I still remember what it was like to have active lupus. Before I got sick I was full of life; I loved to play tennis, ski, and hike in the mountains in all kinds of weather. Then everything changed. My whole body ached and I became tired and lifeless. The fatigue was the symptom that bothered me the most. It was not an ordinary fatigue. It was a drained feeling, a lethargy that did not improve with rest and relaxation; it absorbed my whole person, physically and emotionally. I was so exhausted I could barely lift my arm to attend to my personal needs. I was pathetic. I would sit down in a chair, and when I wanted to get up I could not. I was so tired, I felt paralyzed. I had to reach for the aspirin bottle, swallow a couple, and then wait for them to take effect. After a while my stomach turned sour. The milk I took to alleviate the distress caused by the aspirin produced diarrhea and abdominal cramps. The doctor found that I was sensitive to milk. I had an intolerance of lactose.

As explained by Dr. Stephen Kaplan in Chapter 6, today more is known about why aspirin is such a useful drug in the treatment of lupus. But in 1953, my dependence on aspirin was puzzling to the physician. My doctor used to ask me, "Why do you think that aspirin is helping you?" and my answer always was, "I don't know, but it does."

No matter how well I felt in the morning, I was liable to collapse a few hours later. I had a morbid feeling that I would always feel too tired to do anything. I was worried that I would never regain my confidence. I never planned ahead or even made a simple appointment for fear that I would not be able to keep it."

And through all this, I looked well—a picture of health. This only made things worse. One day I could hear the children talking in the backyard. Leaning out the window, I heard Sara, a seven-year-old neighbor's child, reveal that her mother had told a neighbor that I was not sick, but lazy. "Your mother is lying," my daughter Ingrid countered.

Her sister Martha, then four or five, flew into a rage. "Your mother is a pickle-face!"

The name suited Mrs. Fletcher. Sara and my girls have remained lifelong friends, but even after all these years, whenever my girls speak of Mrs. Fletcher, they still call her "Mrs. Pickle-face," for they have never forgotten or forgiven her indiscretion.

My doctor, too, did not know what to make of my extraordinary sense of fatigue. In those years, physicians were not aware that fatigue could be related directly to the disease. And all I could do was wonder if I was to be stuck forever with this problem.

Dr. Naomi Rothfield believes that fatigue in lupus patients is clearly related to the disease, since it is present prior to the onset of therapy. In most lupus patients, she says, fatigue disappears after the other manifestations of the disease disappear during corticosteroid therapy.

Dr. Rothfield stresses that patients with lupus should be questioned about the presence or absence of fatigue, and that an attempt should be made to evaluate whether fatigue is more or less intense. Most patients are able to recognize the fatigue of the disease, she says, and to distinguish this from the fatigue felt by normal individuals. Dr. Rothfield notes that, in some patients, the onset of fatigue is seen prior to the onset of such disease activities as joint pains or rashes.

Besides fatigue, I was developing a score of queer symptoms that were debilitating and difficult to explain. I had pains in my legs from the knees down, and they felt heavy, as though stuffed with cement. The balls of my feet were constantly inflamed and painful. Regardless of what kind of shoes I wore, my feet hurt. Before getting sick, I was able to walk on the beach or work in my garden barefooted, but now walking on my bare feet was like stepping in fire. My fingertips were red or blue and tender, and very often my palms and the tissue around the base of the nails would look red and tender. I was losing my hair, and my fear of getting bald was growing with every handful. The doctors did not know if the loss of hair was caused by steroids or by the underlying general condition. I also had subcutaneous nodules under my elbows and sometimes on my fingers, but whenever I went to see the doctor the symptoms disappeared. He of course had some difficulty responding to a symptom that had vanished. Thus, discouraged and weary, and also afraid of making myself look ridiculous, I stopped explaining my bizarre symptoms. Watching the doctor's expression change from attentiveness to skepticism convinced me that my explanations were in vain.

I went to see my ophthalmologist because I started having problems with my eyes. My right eye felt as though it were an empty socket. Both eyelids were swollen with fluids, and I could not focus. My vision was blurred most of the time, and on some days I saw double. But when I went to see the ophthalmologist, a myopic man who examined my eyes with the patience of Job, he declared that he wished his eyes were as good as mine. My throat hurt all the time. I had a hard time describing the sensation; first my throat hurt, then it did not. Upon examination the doctor could find no redness or inflammation. "It's clean as a whistle," he said with some amusement. By now, he knew that all my symptoms vanished in his presence.

The first lupus patient I met told me she had suddenly blanked out, did not know who or where she as. The blackouts did not last very long, but they were followed by blinding headaches that did not wane even when she took large doses of codeine. I was fortunate—lupus did not affect my brain. My thinking was clear, I was alert, and I could read. It would be impossible to overestimate the role that reading played in my life. I read and read and read. I was always a reader, and a good book still brought me enormous satisfaction. I read every book by Henry James, the French and Russian classics. I read Mishima and John Cheever. I read fairy tales. I read anything I could find that could hold my attention—philosophy and verse, each volume carrying me over a surprising sequence of crises. I absorbed the poems of Verlaine and Baudelaire, filled my mind and my imagination with thoughts and images from which I drew the strength I needed for survival, and from which I would draw later some of my resources for writing.

My husband was usually optimistic. He believed that I would get well, and he encouraged me to be patient and not to get discouraged. "That's not like you," my husband often said. "You and I have seen many examples of what strength of will, directed toward an objective, can achieve. Remember when you left Bulgaria? You were the last person to leave the country after the German occupation. You went around the world in time of war, because you were determined to come to the United States. When I received your cable from Vladivostok, I was stunned. I didn't know how you got there or how you were going to leave the place. Now you have a new challenge! You must get well!"

What a fantastic trip that long journey to America had been. I left Sofia on March 3, 1941, three days after the German occupation. The borders of Bulgaria were closed, and the only open gate left was the Black Sea. In Varna, I boarded a Russian ship called the *Swanetia*. My parents were not allowed to leave Sofia after the Germans occupied the city. The only person to see me off was a gypsy who carried my luggage from the train station. He was the only one to wish me to "travel in a good hour."

As I stood halfway up the gangplank of the *Swanetia*, I started crying. I was still asking myself, "Should I leave my parents at such a time?" We had had many talks about it, and they thought I should. They urged me to leave. I felt a unique sadness. The final moments of anxiety preceding the departure and the separation from all I had known were full of desperation. The gypsy did not leave me until the last moment. He was waving from the dock as the *Swanetia* pulled its anchors aweigh for the crossing of the Black Sea.

Two days later we docked in Odessa. What a shock that was! I had never seen so many people dressed in rags, so many beggars, so many houses in need of repair, and so many human eyes so full of despair. It was incredible. The Communists had been in power since 1917, and now, twenty-five years later, seeing a sight like this did not make sense. Huddled in my parka, I walked through the streets of Odessa observing the passers-by and wondering if they were the same people I had read about in Dostoevski's novels. People were staring at me too. Very few travelers had been allowed to enter Russia since the Great Revolution, and even fewer had been seen in Odessa. People marveled at my traveling to the New World by myself. I left Odessa six weeks before the Germans demolished the city and thousands of innocent people were killed. I reached Kiev and Moscow. Moscow was another matter. The subways were a sight of wonder: I was afraid to step on the electric escalators, and I was dazzled by the shiny marble, the beautifully painted walls, and the brilliant lights. Red Square and the sights of the city were like pictures from my history books in school. After a week there, I boarded the Trans-Siberian Express, and fifteen days later I arrived in Vladivostok. From there I cabled my husband, who was then my fiancé.

I had to stay for weeks in this forsaken city until I could secure passage to Japan. I crossed the Yellow Sea on the *Makutsu-Maru*, a fifty-year-old ship that carried us over on her last breath. At night I had to stuff blankets in the cracks of my cabin walls to stop the splashing waves from soaking my bed. Half-sinking and half-sailing, the *Makutsu-Maru* saw us safely to Tsuruga in time to see the cherry trees in bloom. Not even in my wildest dreams could I conceive of such beauty. And then the islands of Hawaii—still another world of flowers, blue seas, and blue sky.

I traveled for nearly three months before I reached San Francisco Bay. I can vividly remember when the *Yavata-Maru* glided under the Golden Gate Bridge. The bridge was lit by thousands of lights, and the waves looked golden, while silvery shadows, like fairies, led the ship to its final destination. In the distance, the city of San Francisco was shrouded in mystery under its blanket of fog. And then the sun rose on the horizon, a burst of fire revealing the splendor of the city and the magnificence of the bay.

I remember the day I stood alone on the pier, feeling homesick and frightened about the unknown ahead of me. The screeching of the seagulls and what little I knew of the English language were jumbled in my head. One did not make any more sense than the other.

The customs officials were kind and helpful in San Francisco. They were concerned with my being young, and traveling alone and not speaking the language. An old inspector with bifocals made arrangements for someone to put me on the train to New York, and then personally sent a telegram to my fiancé telling him when to expect me. This was so different from Russia, where they confiscated some of my books—two by Dostoevski—because they were considered to be decadent; or from Japan, where people were hostile because of the prevailing prewar mood; or from Bulgaria, where I was told that I could not take two coats out of the country. I foolishly chose to keep my pink tweed spring coat and let them have my winter one.

Remembering those times stirred up emotions and a vague feeling of confidence. A decision to do something about my health took shape during those moments. I began thinking of selling the huge house in West Newton, Massachusetts, and moving to a smaller place where I could manage with less effort and where the children could walk to school and my husband could walk to the train station. I envisioned a place with less brass to polish, and where I would depend less on hired help. Pursuing those thoughts, I walked into another dream, a dream in which I changed my whole way of life and found a sense of normality within the abnormalities of my disease.

In the following months, while my illness grew progressively worse, I knew that I could not go on living without making some changes. Even if my health improved, living in such a big house would mean constant dependency on outside help, and I had concerns about my family. I was worried that if my illness eventually took me away from them, they should be able to manage by themselves. But these thoughts I kept to myself.

Looking back over my experiences with lupus, I believe that it has constituted an unusual human experience that instilled in me not only a sense of balance, but also a commitment to balance in my life.

When I told my doctor that I was seriously considering selling our house and moving into a smaller place, he asked me what my husband thought about that. "We haven't discussed it yet," I said. "He will need time to get used to the idea!"

"I wouldn't be in a great hurry to sell the house," he said. "Sometimes a patient with symptoms like yours suddenly feels better for unexplained reasons." But I had made up my mind, and I was determined to go through with my plan.

The thought of telling my husband about selling our house horrified me. For him, the place had become a symbol, the planting of his roots in America; it was an anchor for his family. In Bulgaria, a house stayed in the family for generations. It was a place not only for the living, but also for the ancestral ghosts to roam in peace.

Our house* was originally built by a prominent Boston Brahmin

---

* Portions of this material appear in some form in *The Sun Is My Enemy*, a personal account of my battle with lupus (Prentice-Hall, 1972).

family with taste and money to lavish on details. The dining room, with French doors opening to a huge greenhouse, sold me the house, though the old English Tudor was desperately in need of repair. We modernized the kitchen and the bathrooms, replaced the heating system, and repaired the tile roof and crumbling Tory chimney. We covered the floors with Kirman carpets and furnished the rooms with furniture and paintings and pottery we bought in Holland. By the time we were ready to move in, the house had a contemporary flair. It offered all amenities and it preserved a sense of timeless elegance. It was a lovely place.

One day, when I was very tired and discouraged, I burst into tears and told my husband that we had to sell the house. He did not take me seriously; he thought the mood would pass. However, after a year of tears and arguing, he reluctantly agreed, and we did sell the house.

I recalled a bright spring day, better suited for working in the garden, when I had gone to see my doctor at Peter Bent Brigham Hospital in Boston (now Brigham and Woman's Hospital). The year was 1957. "Your lupus is raging," the doctor had said, "and your kidneys are severely damaged. They have collapsed over 60 percent. The prognosis is poor but not hopeless." The doctor's eyes remained on me, but there had been no indication that he wanted to tell me more.

"Am I going to die?" I asked, in a low voice.

"I can't answer that," the doctor said. "Sometimes the damage to the kidneys can reverse itself. I wish I knew how to remove the insulting agent, which in your case is lupus. Unfortunately, we don't have any cure for lupus—not yet, anyhow."

By now, the doctor's pale face looked crimson. It matched the flamboyant red vest he frequently sported under his otherwise conservative tweed jacket. He moved his bulky six-foot-six-inch frame uncomfortably in the black Harvard chair, then rose to his feet. Picking up the vials of blood he had drawn from my arm, he stuck them in the upper pocket of his jacket. His hands were large and steady. I was always aware of them when he drew blood from my arm. "I'll pack some of this blood in dry ice and fly it to the Rockefeller Institute of Medical Research in New York," the doctor said. "At the Rockefeller they have developed a more sensitive way of checking the serum protein. Let's wait until we hear from them. In the meantime, we'll increase the dose of cortisone, and see if it helps."

"Is there any hope?" My voice was a reflex of some inner feelings.

"There is always hope," he answered with a hopeless shrug of his shoulders. "Sometimes the disease can go into a remission, but we have no reliable documentation about that."

I sensed desperation in his efforts to modify the grim reality of the disease. "I can't die! I don't want to die," I wanted to tell him, but my mouth and throat were dry and constricted. As I listened to the doctor's footsteps fade in the hall, my chest felt strangely empty and the emptiness spread through my entire body. Only moments before, I had been a living person; now, this had suddenly changed. The illusory concept of death became strangely real.

On my way to the parking lot, many questions came into my mind, not related to my illness, but to an emerging search for meaning. Why was I born? Why did I get lupus? And why was I going to die so young? Why did I get married, have children, go to school, and have so many dreams and aspirations?

When I reached my car, the parking lot attendant smiled. "It's a beautiful day, Miss," he said. "Not a cloud in the sky." I stared. I was not aware of the sky, and his face looked out of shape and terribly distorted.

On Route 9, I was startled by the appearance of the houses, buses, cars, and lurid greens of the trees. Somehow nothing seemed real. It was like another world. I drove automatically. I passed by a vegetable stand selling pink potted geraniums. The flowers became confused in my mind with the flamingos I had seen in Florida when I first developed lupus. Then I drove past a rambling brick house with white curtains in the windows. The house was surrounded by bright green grass, lilac trees in bloom, and white birches. It looked like my parents' house, where I grew up in Bulgaria. "The house is gone," I muttered to myself. It had been demolished in the war. When I was small, my mother told me stories about her childhood, about my Grandmother Maya, and Great-Grandmother Henrietta, whose name and looks and stubbornness I have inherited. My mother's stories had made me feel part of a long life that had no beginning and no end. "But Mother is dead," I heard my voice in the empty car. "We are all dead! Everybody is dead, but they don't know it!"

Life and death were jumbled in my head, and one made no more sense than the other.

When I arrived home my children came running toward me. "Mommy, Mommy, look! Martha can tie her shoes!" Martha, who was three and a half, was waving a small brown shoe, beaming with pride, "Leave me alone!" I screamed. "I am dizzy. I am sick, I can't listen to this noise!" Startled by my rudeness, the children became quiet. I glanced at Martha. A more pathetic face could hardly be imagined. She was holding onto her shoe, sobbing, and she looked smaller than she actually was. I picked her up and gathered her tightly in my arms. In contrast to all the previous distortions, her tearful face looked real. "Show me how you can tie your shoes," I said, wiping her tears. Watching her tiny fingers making a perfect bow, I felt as though the hollow in my chest was filling up with love. "You learn so fast," I said, holding back my tears, "but there is so much more for you to learn. You've got a long way to go yet . . . I'll be here to help you with every moment I'll be around. I'll make an effort. I promise you I'll try."

Until that day I had felt that if I could not be well, death might be better than living. But now, no matter how sick I was, I wanted to stay alive, not only for my sake, but also for the sake of my children.

In the weeks and months that followed, I flowed with the disease. I was open to emotions and self-examination before I undertook a basic self-reeducation in order to survive the tribulations of the illness. I developed a stern discipline, making an effort hour by hour and living a day at a time. In the passage of those years I had to accept not only the disease but also that this was life, and one must live it.

Dr. Rene Dubos, from the Rockefeller Institute, in his book entitled *The Torch of Life: Continuity in Living Experience*, writes that adaptation and conscious effort are important to one's survival. Every person, he says, has reserves of a wide range of potentialities, which often remain unexpressed. Anyone, with a little systematic effort, becomes better at almost any kind of work and more resistant to any kind of stress. In the final analysis, the potential of human beings becomes actualized through the process of meeting challenges with a creative spirit. History, Dr. Dubos says, teaches that human beings without effort are sure to deteriorate; and humans cannot progress without effort, they cannot be happy without effort. I have thought often about that.

In the spring of 1958, we bought a new house a few miles away from where we had lived. The new house was located on a hill and was surrounded by huge white birches, oaks, and beech trees. It was very pleasant. As I was gathering some strength to move, my husband bought the old house back and rented it to the buyers with an option to buy it in a year if we were to stay in the new house. I did not panic. I was sure that he would get used to the new place. And I thought all would be well.

Shortly after we moved, I grew stronger, I grew healthier, and I was getting back my old sense of peace and self-reliance. I was like a new person. My husband could not believe the change that was taking place in me. I approached each day with a sense of joy. With the help of a highschool girl, I began planting flowers. I had an urge to be close with nature and dig in the soil. On a deeper level I was seeking to establish a relationship of meaning, a feeling of trust in the multiple realities of life. In my new house, I felt less lonely and less isolated because the windows were floor-to-ceiling, and I could look out on my garden and the open sky. I could lie in bed and watch the moonlight creep across my flowers, and the snow falling over my trees. No one could know if my remission was prompted by treatment or by natural causes. But never could I have hoped for such a recovery. However, I harbored no false hopes; I knew that I was not cured. No cure existed. The lupus could recur at any time, but the nightmare was over for the time being, and I could now hope based on this experience. At the time I had no idea that my remission would last for over thirty-two years, that I would never need to take any more medications and that all my tests would be consistently negative. I had no idea that someday I would write books and stories about lupus, start a national lupus foundation, and travel all over the world to help others.

After my remission had lasted for several years, I went back to Europe and met my Bulgarian doctor, Professor Liuben Popoff, in Lyon. He asked me what had kept me going when I had active lupus. "I don't know," I said. "Perhaps my spirit didn't break down completely. Perhaps it is genetic," I mused. "My mother had a will of iron."*

"This might have helped more than you think," he answered.

---

* Parts of the conversation with Professor Popoff appear in *The Sun Is My Enemy*, Prentice-Hall, 1972.

"The will to live can help the medical treatment to work. The physician's spirit is reinforced by a brave patient. The physician searches for allies. He first looks to the patient, I am sure. Your American doctor must have found strength in your spirit. And you, you must have trusted him and drawn strength from his effort, intelligence, and dedication. Is that not so?" And then he asked the question other lupus patients have asked me over the years. "And now, what do you do to stay well?"

I told him that somehow I emerged from all this helped by a feeling of hope. Perhaps that, too, is a genetic gift. I told him that I am reinforcing an old medical maxim called Osler's aphorism: "If you want to live a long life, get a chronic disease and take care of it." However, some days when the sunshine is beautiful, when it brings happy feelings to everyone, I look out and feel saddened. I want to bask in the sun, I want to forget that the sun is my enemy. At such times I tell myself that I must make peace with the disease and accept it as part of living. Until then, there will be times of unnecessary anger, disappointment, and fear.

In my case the support of my family was crucial in carrying me through the endless days and months of pain and frustrations. Recovery from lupus was slow. Continual surveillance by the physician was needed at every step in order to help me meet physical emergencies and emotional and psychological stresses. Few therapies are really effective in lupus, and patients are helped mainly by interaction with the physician and the alleviation of symptoms. I was treated with every treatment known to science in 1953. However, the things that I remember best are not the medications that my doctor prescribed, but what he taught me about my body and about my disease. My doctor wanted me to know and accept all that was to be known about lupus. He felt that this was important, and indeed the knowledge that I gained helped me to defend myself against misapprehensions and unnecessary fears. It also helped me to avoid situations that could affect my illness and make it worse. Once I was able to understand my limits and to acknowledge them to myself, I could more easily explain them to my family and enlist their help.

My doctor was always the person who could help me, and I was the person who needed his help. In his presence I could talk about my emotions and how I was spending my days. No longer was I learning about the disease alone. He was learning, as well, about my illness.

To the doctor, lupus represents laboratory measurements and organ dysfunctions, while to me the dysfunction of my kidneys meant pain, nausea, dizziness, and fluid retention. It also meant fear and the anticipation of further complications as well as the horror of possible death.

What can a physician do to help the lupus patient, from the patient's point of view? The most important factor is communication. The patient must trust the physician. The physician can earn that trust by asking the patient all the things that bother him or her, and then explaining what those symptoms and signs mean. As Dr. Peter Schur, director of lupus research at Brigham and Women's Hospital in Boston says, it means listening and explaining. Many patients are fearful of bringing up sensitive subjects such as sex, marital tensions, and financial problems. Patients appreciate being able to discuss these things with someone they can trust, and whose counsel and advice they respect. This trust facilitates good medical management, and it can only be earned over a period of time.

The following chapters discuss some of the problems unique to the lupus patient. While the health-care team can be extremely helpful in some of these situations, others may require the special assistance of marriage counselors, lawyers, or other qualified professionals. Living with lupus can be difficult, but with increasing public awareness of this illness and advances in many different fields of research, we can only hope that many of the obstacles before us will soon be overcome.

12

Lupus and Marriage

What are some of the marital tensions that develop for lupus patients, and what can physicians do about them? As I have stressed before, a major problem is that many patients look relatively well, even though they may feel ill and uncomfortable. Family members and spouses see what appears to be a relatively well person who complains about feeling ill and fatigued and may be unable to assume his or her share of normal household responsibilities or hold down a job. The patient will, if asked, says Dr. Peter Schur, tell how difficult it is to explain these problems to close family members. Marriage counselors may be helpful, but the physician who is aware of the varied manifestations of lupus can also play a vital role in the patient's well-being. The physician can help by explaining the disease and its manifestations, not only to the patient, but also to the family. Obviously, says Dr. Schur, some patients have other reasons for these complaints that do not necessarily relate to lupus. Some people are chronic complainers; some are simply depressed. But they all need help, regardless.

Tension often arises in young people about to be married, revolving around concerns about having children. Many young women, despite changing social mores, feel that they are not whole persons, and are inadequate wives, if they cannot have children with their spouses. Patients with lupus may need to be counseled to delay pregnancy until the disease activity subsides somewhat. "But the doctor should give hope to the patient that, in many cases, this simmering down will happen," says Dr. Schur. And it does.

Financial difficulties can be an enormous headache. Many young couples who marry these days assume two incomes, and plan accordingly, for example, to buy a house. Couples must be helped to develop a realistic point of view, not just about lupus, but also about life. Blame should be avoided. The patient may want to consider a part-time job, rather than full-time work. The physician can provide job references that downplay the stigma of having the disease. In cases involving incapacitation, physicians can help patients apply for Social Security Disability. This issue will be discussed in Chapter 16, which shows how the letter the doctor writes plays a major role in helping the patient to get Social Security Disability.

Patients often have difficulty speaking about sex to their doctors. This is a serious problem that nobody likes to talk about, including patients, spouses, and doctors.

The divorce rate is high among lupus patients, and many have told me that sex plays a role in this drama. The woman patient senses the spouse's need for sexual gratification, but in her drained state she cannot always be the charming and fulfilling partner she was in the past. The spouse feels unfairly denied. He is healthy, with healthy urges, and, although he might not talk about it in the beginning, the woman fears that he will eventually become open about it, which certainly may happen. This is very frightening to a woman who has lost her vitality and looks, and who, at such times, needs the affection and the care of her spouse or friend. Many women make the mistake of thinking that it is she who is depriving her spouse, when the culprit is really her illness. Some become desperate and begin to resent the husband whose life they have complicated.

Patients complain that physicians are more than willing to discuss their physical problems with sex and to give them prescriptions for ointments and medications, but very few have been able to help with the more complex psychological problems. One patient told me that, even in remission, she needed a physician's help. She had sublimated her sexual feelings for long stretches of time, so that healthy urges and desires were deeply buried. Another patient told how, while she was in remission, her husband became hostile and resentful. The sexual energy that he had repressed while waiting for her to be well again was suddenly released in anger and violence. She wished she were ill again, rather than have to cope with such a new and painful situation. Physicians say that the majority of

patients do not want to speak about sex because they have developed
a dishonesty about it. Patients feel that physicians ought to help
them to discuss the problem.

I spoke with a patient whose story reflects the experiences of many
other patients. This is what she said.

> My husband is a vigorous man. He enjoys sex and is a
> happy person by nature. I, too, was like that. Our marriage
> was great until I got lupus. Now I have gained over forty
> pounds from the steroids; I look grotesque. I have lost most
> of my hair; it comes out in bunches and I seldom comb it
> anymore. I look in the mirror and I don't recognize myself.
> It is like staring at a stranger. My personality is changing
> too. I am growing increasingly frustrated by the limitations
> this strange illness is placing on me. Dangers, real and
> imaginary, trouble me all the time. I am very depressed.
> My whole being, every living part of me, has been involved
> in this depression, and there is no one who can under-
> stand—no one who can help me. I thought my husband
> understood and accepted things as they are, but he has
> changed too! The tension between us is constant, and it
> increases before we go to bed at night. Lying in bed, so
> close to one another, increases our nervousness. We don't
> talk of our fears or true feelings for each other anymore.
> Even when we make love, we do so with less trust in one
> another. We don't know how to relate to one another any-
> more. I suspect that he resents my illness, my bloated body,
> my exhaustion, and my loss of interest in sex.
> My husband tells me that I am thinking constantly about
> my illness. I thought of nothing else. I can't help it! I wish
> that I could scream at him for not understanding, but I can
> only turn my face away so he can't see my eyes filling up
> with tears. I can't help worrying. It breaks my heart that I
> am not much of a wife to him. Whenever he wants to make
> love, I am tired. I feel fatigued to the point where I don't
> have the strength to turn over from one side to the other.
> I have lost my spontaneity; I have lost my interest in sex.
> My husband still expects me to be dynamic in bed and show
> him a good time. I try to please him, but there is no fun
> in tired sex. My husband tells me that I am tired because
> I do too much. I have to take it easy, he says, I have to
> spare myself. He goes on and on . . . He keeps repeating

the same words over and over. It is a constant reminder—
more like a constant complaint.

Actually, it is just the reverse. I do less and less every
day. I can't do anything, in fact. That is how it is now—I
barely manage to change the beds and clean the bathroom.
My husband flares out in rage when I contradict him or try
to explain. I realize with sadness that he, like everyone else,
cannot understand what's going on in my soul; the degree
of guilt I am experiencing is great, and it adds to an already
great burden. It is hard for me to forgive myself for my
irritation, and for denying him sexual satisfaction. And I
myself have to do without these pleasures, which makes it
even more difficult.

Night after night, I lie beside him, tense, and listen to
his powerful chest breathing forth the torment of my illness
and our despair. Some nights, in the middle of a restless
sleep, he calls my name, perhaps looking for the girl he
married. And I murmur the same words over and over,
"Dear God, don't let him stop loving me." Hideous thoughts
flash through my mind. I fear that he is going to divorce
me. I have never felt so lonely in my entire life. I listen to
the silence of my soul and search for what is left of me, so
I can pull myself together!

The following is an excerpt from a story written by a young nurse,
Molly Page, who is also a lupus patient:*

This is the story of my marriage, which lasted about four
years. Its personal and one-sided observations reflect some
of my feelings.

I do not want to be unfair to my former husband (especially since this is my side of the story and not his), but we
both had numerous faults.

We had two main difficulties. The first was a problem
with communication—a common complaint in this day and
age (1981). Possibly, if we had more time together we would
eventually have worked this problem of noncommunication
out?? Most likely, this is just wishful thinking on my part.

Second, we had sexual difficulties—which may have
stemmed initially from my disability and difficulty in move-

---

* Molly Page, R.N., is president of the Lupus Foundation of Virginia.

ment. This was a very emotional experience for me. It was compounded by our communication problems.

At first I thought that maybe I could learn different positions for sex (to make it less painful for me), and thereby reduce my husband's anxiety. I talked to my physician about this problem. Most of his advice was to read a book on the subject (of which there have been numerous volumes filled). It seems like no matter what I tried my husband always said that he was "afraid of hurting me." I tried to remedy this by taking pain medication an hour or two before bed, but this was to no avail.

The next hurdle was birth control. Because an exacerbation of SLE symptoms was precipitated (in my case) by the use of oral contraceptives, we resorted to using other methods of birth control. It seems like everything I used was not spontaneous enough for my husband. His favorite excuse was that he was too tired—I thought that was supposed to be my excuse. This only tended to make me feel responsible for most problems (sexual or not).

I can remember crying myself to sleep during those times; possibly this may have been caused by my feelings of inadequacy and frustration, by drug therapy, by the disease itself, or by a combination of these factors. Regardless of the etiology, I felt miserable.

And later in her story, Molly writes:

My husband and I separated in October of 1977. A little over a year later we were divorced.

I realize that my being sick put a lot of stress on both of us. I spent most of my first few years of marriage in the hospital. Therefore, we never had that so-called important first year of marriage. My husband was attending a local university, plus he had a part-time job in the hospital. In addition he was trying to keep our marriage together (which must have been a difficult task since I was in the hospital most of the time). This rationalization may be a defense mechanism—to try to relieve myself of guilt. We thought that when he graduated from college there would be a lessening of pressure. This did not occur. Subsequently, we decided to try separation for a while. Eventually, this led to a divorce.

Even though the divorce was by mutual consent, I still felt responsible for causing it. It is ridiculous to feel disappointed in yourself because divorce can (and does) happen to anybody.

I still think of my former husband. Naturally there are some fond memories, and we are not bitter toward one another (at least there are no bad feelings on my part). I do miss him, but the feelings of guilt are gradually subsiding—it is now 1981.

About a year after my divorce, I had my name changed. I realize that I should have done this when I was divorced, but I think that I wanted to hold on to some part of my former husband, even if it was only his name. Perhaps retaining the name gave me some kind of hope that we would eventually get back together.

At any rate, divorce is *not* the end of the world, even though it seems like it at the time. Naturally, some permanent psychological scars remain, but they are only scars—not open sores. Regardless of how much one loved her husband, the pain *will* gradually subside. This may take a number of years. It is important to remember that *love* is an ambiguous term, in that various people define it in different ways according to their individual needs. I am no expert on divorce—by any means. But like most things in life one has to experience it before one can really empathize with others, although this is a difficult way to learn. Unfortunately, most things in life are discovered in this manner.

In my opinion, health-care professionals should be taught something about sexual problems. It took me a long time to bring the subject up with my physician (probably because of the stigma attached plus my own embarrassment). Then he was reluctant to talk about it (possibly embarrassment on his part). The stigma about sex is slowly disappearing, and there are now some courses that can be taken at the college level. I hope that this stigma will cease to exist in the future. I think that there is currently a generation gap regarding sex. Each generation now seems a little more open to discuss sexual problems.

Many couples will face communication and/or sexual problems. With any luck these difficulties may be worked out. In some cases, the problems may ultimately lead to a divorce.

It was not unusual for us to have to face communication and sexual difficulties. The additional problems imposed by my prolonged illness and the intervening problems ultimately led to our breakup. A marriage without the complications of a chronic illness is at best difficult. *Both* partners have to really work on their relationship for it to succeed.

There is no way of knowing whether we could have worked through our problems. The imposition of my illness made this literally impossible. Counseling might have helped if we had tried it (this is purely conjecture on my part). The social stigma attached to any kind of counseling is also disappearing with time. I think that counseling may be helpful in that there is an objective (unrelated) third party. This is probably part of the "nurse" speaking.

It is easy to rationalize intellectually the combination of factors that may cause a marriage to fail. But emotionally this rationalization often falls apart. Time seems to be the only real remedy (cure).

Statistics show that over half of all marriages in which one of the spouses has lupus fail (although I suspect that this would happen in any marriage where one of the partners is chronically ill).

Possibly, eventually the psychological (mental and behavioral) causes of divorce will be solved.

Lupus patients are often given tranquilizers to allay anxiety and other emotional problems caused by some aspects of the disease. Physicians* believe that some of these drugs, on occasion, suppress orgasm. They also believe that cortisone, a drug often used in the treatment of lupus, presents a host of side effects. (Medications used in the treatment of lupus have been discussed in Chapter 6; some, however, are appropriate to mention in connection with sex.) Patients who are taking cortisone bruise more easily, and in some cases can develop a painful hip condition known as avascular necrosis, which can create pain when they are having intercourse. Cortisone,

* Sheldon P. Blau, M.D., "Sex and Systemic Lupus Erythematosus," in "Living and Loving," Arthritis Foundation, 1982.

when used regularly, can create sexual apathy for some. Others claim that cortisone stimulates their energy and their desire for sex.

Some patients believe that their sexual problem is unique, not realizing that other patients have the same concerns; other patients feel that nothing can be gained by talking with another person about it. Yet only when patients realize that their sexual problems have also been experienced by other individuals will they find understanding and help. I do not believe that all lupus patients have problems with their sex lives, but I am convinced that it is not uncommon.

I spoke with Dr. Theodore Nadelson and asked him for his thoughts on this subject. Dr. Nadelson stressed that it is best for both partners to accept that the problem of lupus exists *between* them. It may be in the patient's body, but it is a problem that must be handled by both marriage partners because it affects their relationship. The sexual act, after all, is an expression of interchange with another person. When it is not desired, it may be because of a sense that the body itself is not worthy of such an interchange. "Lupus is a disease that afflicts young people," says Dr. Nadelson, "particularly women. They are in the generative, youthful, and libidinal portion of their lives, and sexuality, if not sex, is very important. The sexual act itself, coitus, does not have to be the purpose or goal of intimate interaction. Sexuality can be expressed in touching, in embracing, and in holding."

For some lupus patients, sexual intercourse, or any kind of overly energetic expression, may be too much. According to Dr. Nadelson, "The partner may be too demanding or the patient too resisting. Both have to adapt, and take into account the limitations and restraints imposed by the facts of lupus. I want to emphasize that mutual pleasure can be given within the limits imposed by the disease. A partner's acceptance of this will begin with the understanding that the disease does set limitations. Reduced sexual ardor should not be interpreted as lack of interest in the other person. Sexual interest may wane, but the need for the other person will continue as before.

"This is not to say that everybody can withstand such difficulties. Young people especially may find them extremely stressful. A husband of a woman physically disabled by lupus, or whose sexual interest has decreased because of it, may question his partner's interest in the relationship, and even his own. At this point, a physician or counselor or psychiatrist may be helpful. I would hope that the physician could act as counselor and sex therapist. Less strenuous ways may be found in which sexual interaction can continue. What is needed is a physician who is not afraid to talk about sex and who is knowledgeable enough to counsel in it.

"I certainly believe that not just the patient, but both partners need counseling on this. In other words, the relationship itself is the subject of discourse. Perhaps the doctor, as a counselor, can discuss the problem with both parties, helping both to understand and appreciate that at times neither may want to have a sexual relationship. That does not have to be the point at which they slip away from each other. Such moments can be times of quiet exchanges, of tenderness, and of an affirmation that the couple is going to get through this together. However, some people still see marriage only as a love relationship. It is wonderful if there is love in the marriage, but marriage has other components too. The family, possibly children, are only one facet of marriage. Most important are all the many intertwining aspects of the relationship that develops over the years between a man and a woman. These, from the point of view of advancing years, are really much more relevant than the physical love that was present in the beginning. Sexual intercourse is not the purpose of marriage, although it is one of its important facets. Lupus—or another disease, for that matter—may even make a marriage stronger and better. I would not recommend the interposition of such a difficult disease for that purpose, but some people do better with it.

"Most people need some kind of counseling, to deal not only with the disease, but with the relationship that is troubled by the disease. For this purpose, I think the internist or the specialist needs to be more than a purveyor of medication. Again, he or she needs to deliver a 'dose of the doctor' along with the medication. And to do that the physician needs to know himself or herself. Perhaps the physician could benefit from some counseling—not for himself or herself alone, but because he or she might be able to help the patient deal more effectively with everyday problems. Such issues sometimes transcend even those monumental ones caused by deficits in the immune system response."

13

Lupus
and Pregnancy

In the past, studies of the relationship between SLE and pregnancy often produced contradictory reports. Depending on the data, pregnancy either affected lupus patients adversely, or had beneficial effects.

Today medical investigators are more knowledgeable about this subject, and guidelines based on current relevant information are essential. This will be helpful to the patients and also to the gynecologists who take care of them.

In my case, every pregnancy ran a different course. With the first pregnancy I had kidney involvement; with the second, I had phlebitis (inflammation of the veins) and ulceration of the veins. The third pregnancy ended in a miscarriage; and with the last pregnancy, I developed purpura (hemorrhage into the tissues) with a very low platelet count. This created a serious problem when the baby was being born. I bled excessively. For a while both the physician and I were in distress. In the late 1940s, I did not know that I had lupus, and my gynecologist was just as ignorant as I was about the disease. But fortunately Dr. Louis Albert was an experienced gynecologist, and with some luck and lots of patience, he pulled me through. With my last child, he did not leave the hospital for forty-eight hours, and I recall his disappointment about missing the Harvard-Yale football game.

When I see my children healthy and well, I count my blessings. They are now parents themselves, and we have five beautiful grandchildren. Would I go through the same experiences again? The answer is yes. However, I would make sure to choose an obstetrician who is familiar with the disease and who could work closely with a lupus specialist. The physicians who take care of lupus patients believe that pregnancy is when the patient needs expert care and extra support, both from the family and from the physician.

When I was pregnant I felt very tired, and during the delivery I felt lifeless. When I see a pregnant lupus patient I remember that, and I can relate to what the woman is going through. I think how important it is, when one expects a child, to feel secure within oneself. I wonder whether the gynecologist is aware of the lupus fatigue and its effects at such crucial moments.

Some patients question whether physicians can predict, from the course of the disease during one pregnancy, how lupus will affect a subsequent pregnancy.

The young lupus patient has many problems and many worries before and after she conceives. Many patients ask about the advisability of pregnancy while their lupus is active. Pregnant women worry about the potent drugs they must take to combat lupus. They worry not only about themselves, but also about their children. They need clear answers about the antimalarial drugs such as chloroquine or hydroxychloroquine (Plaquenil), the steroids, azothioprine (Imuran), cyclophosphamide (Cytoxan), the tranquilizers, and other potent medications.

Patients with high blood pressure or nephritis (inflammation of the kidneys) worry about becoming pregnant and about what pregnancy will do to alter the long-term course of their illness. Some ask whether an abortion poses a threat to the lupus patient's life and want to know when an abortion is recommended. Patients who are told that they will have to deliver by cesarean section want to know if they are at greater risk during this or any other surgical procedure. And still others want to know if they should wait for a period of remission before becoming pregnant, or if patients with mild disease conceive more readily than those with more active disease. Once pregnant, women have such concerns as:

"Will I be able to breast feed?"

"Will I be able to take care of my child adequately?"

"Will my child develop lupus?"

"Will my child have a predisposition to the disease?"

"Will I be able to cope with the lupus fatigue during this crucial time of my life?"

Dr. Robert B. Zurier, professor of medicine and chief of rheumatology at the University of Pennsylvania Medical School, has written extensively on the subject of lupus and pregnancy and is currently involved in lupus research. Dr. Zurier is particularly interested in the role of prostaglandins (substances that can act as hormones, vitamins, or enzymes) in immune responses. These compounds appear to be especially important in regulating blood pressure and blood clotting in pregnancy. Dr. Zurier takes care of many lupus patients, and he is keenly aware of the patient's need for straightforward information on lupus and pregnancy. He responded to many of these questions:

"Once thought to be ill advised, marriage and pregnancy can now be considered by nearly all young women with systemic lupus erythematosus. Concerns persist, however, and the special risks (these must be considered high-risk pregnancies) associated with pregnancy must be understood by the patient and her husband. One concern—a surprise to me when brought to my attention by Mrs. Aladjem—is that some SLE patients still believe that pregnancy is out of the question for them, and they think they are advised they can conceive because the physician is interested in studying them. Most SLE patients can be assured that motherhood is a very real possibility for them. If the patient continues to feel like a guinea pig, then further advice should be sought from other physicians and health-care workers, and from other SLE patients.

"As a group, SLE patients are no less fertile than the general population. Of course, disease activity and/or corticosteroid treatment can temporarily alter the menstrual cycle, preventing pregnancy for a time. Since fertility is not a problem, contraception is an issue to be addressed. Birth-control pills do not induce lupus or abnormal laboratory tests in normal women, and they probably do not make lupus worse, since many SLE patients take birth-control pills and do quite well. However, chronic administration of oral contraceptives is associated with an increased incidence of hypertension, blood clots, and strokes, probably by inducing some change in blood-vessel walls. Since a basic problem in SLE is often inflammation at the blood-vessel walls, the most prudent decision for the patient would be to use other forms of contraception. The safest would be a condom or a diaphragm with spermicidal jelly. Intrauterine devices (IUDs) seem to cause more trouble (bleeding, infection) for SLE patients than they do for other young women.

"There are two sides to the SLE-pregnancy coin: the effect of pregnancy on SLE, and the effect of SLE on pregnancy and the fetus."

EFFECT OF PREGNANCY ON SLE

"Patients with lupus do not necessarily do worse during pregnancy, but renal disease in particular can get worse. Naturally, the course of disease is the most favorable if the patient is in remission at the time of conception. However, since the *duration* of remission has no relation to the course of disease during pregnancy, it is not necessary to wait a prolonged and arbitrary period of time after onset of remission to undertake pregnancy. This is especially important for those patients who have delayed marriage and pregnancy. Patients should not think that their course during one pregnancy predicts how they will fare during subsequent pregnancies. Thus, one course may be stormy, the next tranquil. Pregnancy does not alter the long-term course of SLE. In fact, lupus patients who have been pregnant have a better prognosis as a group than patients who do not become pregnant. That is probably because patients with milder disease more often become pregnant.

"Motherhood will of course place increased physical and psychological demands on the lupus patient, and she must be prepared to deal with them. The patient's energy will be sorely taxed, and undue exertion may lead to a flare in disease activity."

EFFECT OF SLE ON PREGNANCY AND THE FETUS

"Miscarriage is high (25–50 percent) for pregnant women with lupus and far exceeds the national average of 15 percent. Surprisingly, the incidence of miscarriage is not related to maternal disease activity. On the other hand, premature birth occurs more often when lupus flares. Fortunately, with better management of SLE patients in general, premature birth is not now a major problem. Similarly, an increase in disease activity characteristic of the early (4–8 weeks) postpartum period has yielded greater awareness of the problem, more intelligent use of corticosteroids, and better overall management of patients. Corticosteroid treatment of the mother does not have an adverse effect on the fetus.

"Although the risk to the SLE patient of losing her baby is substantial, the chances of having a normal child are very high, and the children develop and mature normally. One qualification must be voiced: Although it is very rare, complete heart block occurs in babies born to SLE mothers far more often than it does in the general population. In this condition, there is damage to the tissues that conduct the signals that keep the heart beating. Again, the condition is very rare, but it must be mentioned."

GENERAL MANAGEMENT

"Combining the experience and judgment of an obstetrician and a physician skilled in caring for lupus patients best serves the needs of a pregnant SLE patient. These two can work together closely to make appropriate decisions during pregnancy and after childbirth. Patients should be sure to obtain sufficient rest and not hesitate to report any aspect of their pregnancy that troubles them. Fatigue, often characteristic of lupus, is magnified during pregnancy. Indeed, the obstetrical team must be aware that the lupus patient in labor may tire more easily than they expect. Vaginal delivery is recommended, and the indications for cesarean section should not be different than for other women."

THERAPY

"Drug therapy presents potential hazards to the developing fetus. If at all possible, aspirin and similar drugs (nonsteroidal antiinflammatory drugs) should not be given to pregnant patients. It is probably best to stop the antimalarial drugs (such as Plaquenil) at onset of pregnancy, even though patients have taken these drugs through their pregnancies and have delivered normal healthy infants.

"So-called immunosuppressive drugs such as Cytoxan and Imuran should be withheld unless the life of the mother is threatened. Although normal babies have been born to mothers taking these drugs, the long-term effects of such drugs on these children are unknown. Thus corticosteroids are the mainstay of treatment for pregnant SLE patients, and vigorous corticosteroid therapy, rather than interruption of pregnancy, is the treatment of choice for flares of disease activity. However, if exacerbation of disease, especially with nephritis, during the first trimester is severe, and if the patient does not respond to treatment, then therapeutic abortion may be considered. Beyond the first trimester every effort must be made to avoid therapeutic abortion. Years ago, mid-trimester abortions were not uncommonly fatal in SLE patients. With better understanding of the disease and its treatment, that is no longer the case. Nonetheless, the procedure carries some risk and should not be undertaken lightly. Since exacerbation of SLE is common soon after delivery, evacuation of the uterus would not by itself be expected to benefit the patient."

BREAST-FEEDING

"A recurring question is whether the SLE patient should breast-feed her child. Breast-feeding demands a considerable amount of the mother's energy, and in some patients might result in undue fatigue. On the other hand, a woman who is comfortable with breast-feeding and who can get appropriate rest should not be discouraged from breast-feeding her infant. A small proportion of whatever drug is administered to the mother will appear in breast milk. However, the amounts are very small. Women taking as much as thirty milligrams per day of prednisone breast-feed their infants without causing noticeable harm. A reasonable procedure for the mother treated with prednisone would be to take the drug in the morning, breast-feed in the morning, bottle-feed late morning and early afternoon, then breast-feed evening and night. Mothers treated with immunosuppressive drugs should not breast-feed their children."

ADOPTION

"SLE patients, just like many other young women, are sometimes not able to conceive, and therefore consider adoption as a means to have a family. Some adoption agencies may not be receptive to this idea. This restrictive, uninformed view is not aimed at SLE patients in particular, but extends to patients with other diseases that are well controlled, and even to people over forty years old. The physician is often in a position to help the patient by outlining carefully to agency officials the nature of SLE and explaining that SLE patients are perfectly good mothers. Reason does not always prevail, but the effort should be made."

CONCLUSIONS

"SLE patients should be encouraged to live full lives. For women, that includes marriage and motherhood if desired. These undertakings, of course, are difficult under the best of circumstances. The SLE patient must be aware of the special problems that may be associated with her pregnancies. Extra support from family and physicians and others responsible for her care is crucial to the pregnant lupus patient."

Dr. Zurier's point concerning adoption is interesting. Recently I spoke to a young lupus patient who was told that she could not have any children because her kidneys were severely damaged. This woman wonders whether her spouse can look ahead to a life with her, but without a growing family. They are considering adopting a child, but they are encountering difficulties with the adoption agency. Many adoption agencies, ignorant of the disease, are reluctant to allow lupus patients to adopt. Such patients need help from physicians, who can explain the nature of the illness to adoption agencies. But do all gynecologists and obstetricians understand how lupus affects a human life? Do they know the effects of pregnancy on the disease? The effects of lupus on pregnancy? And do they know how to manage the patient during and after pregnancy? Are they adequately prepared to meet the emotional needs of the patients during such trying times?

One of the most outspoken advocates for educating physicians about lupus is Dr. Naomi Rothfield, a professor of medicine at the University of Connecticut School of Medicine. Dr. Rothfield is the chairperson of the department of rheumatology and is a renowned medical investigator and clinician who has much compassion for the lupus patient. Stressing that lupus involves symptoms and signs of many different parts of the body, frequently at different times, Dr. Rothfield says that many of her patients are young women who go to their family physician or gynecologist when their first symptoms of lupus appear. Dr. Rothfield says that those physicians frequently either cannot treat the disease or do not know how to diagnose it, and some, she says, tend to belittle the complaints of the patient, because, in the beginning of the disease, they can find no physical abnormalities on examination.

Guilt and uncertainties are the patient's constant companions. They want to understand not only their physical stresses, but also their emotional reactions. They need help to relieve the anxiety associated with these uncertainties and fears during this important time in their lives.

14

Lupus in Men

The clinical profiles of males with lupus are essentially the same as those of females, and the psychosocial problems are difficult to manage for both sexes.

Adding another dimension to the problems of the male patient is the fact that lupus is described in the lay literature as a disease of young women. One often sees a definition of lupus in a dictionary that reads, "Fatal disease of young women," and some medical dictionaries describe lupus as a generalized disorder affecting mainly middle-aged women.

The wife of a male patient from Detroit* wrote the following lines:

> Lupus is usually diagnosed among young women of child-bearing age. How many times do we all hear or read this statement . . . or a variation of it! Although the statement is essentially true, I wonder how many of us have stopped to consider its effect on the male lupus patient. . . . For a married man with children, the need to "prove" himself has been satisfied before lupus became severe. It is the young male lupus patient who is still subject to the intense "peer" pressures at a time when being different in any way is particularly undesirable. . . . There is nothing written about

* An excerpt from an article written by Nancy Hubbard, published by The Michigan Lupus Foundation.

the need to create self-confidence and to avoid identity problems.

And a male patient wrote:

I would like to point out that all the publicity about lupus is slanted toward women. I am not a male chauvinist, but I resent the fact that it is rare that SLE is spoken about in terms of men!

I would like to point out that since 1976 I started having problems—going from doctor to doctor, to be told, as many other lupus patients have, it's all in your head. You talk about self-esteem, ego, morale, value, sexual needs, and how they will affect housekeeping and mothering! Well, let's talk about how it affects men for a change!

How we can keep our wives and children happy and fulfill their needs as well as ours? How do I as a "broken man" tell my two-year-old child that Daddy can't play with her, walk with her, play in the sun with her, or quite often, communicate with her?!!!!

I'm having trouble accepting all the articles I read that are directed only to women. I've had problems with the medical profession and the Social Security system—probably more so because I am a man!!

Not until 1978–79, when my wife rushed me to the emergency room at the hospital and my doctor put me in intensive care, did I start to get minor results. Finally in 1979 my doctor wanted to give me more antibiotics to lower my blood count, which was quite elevated! I refused to take any additional medication until they read my critique, which was taken from all my hospital stays. I underlined the high points after my wife typed up four pages condensing my medical history. Then and only then was a proper course of action taken. It has been one year since I've been put on a steroid program; finally I'm down to prednisone every other day, but I have not had a remission period. I must take quite a bit of medication: Minipress, 4 mg daily; Lasix, 20 mg daily; Tranxene, 22.5 mg daily; amitriptyline, 50 to 100 mg daily; nitroglycerin as needed; Tedral for asthma as needed; Imodium as needed; Tylenol #3 as needed!! Plus constant infections where antibiotics are necessary!! My resident shrink tells me I handle my disease well, but he's not in my shoes;

he's not feeling the emptiness, torment, inadequacies, memory losses, and stuttering that continue to make me want to withdraw into my own little world!!

The best thing I've learned about this disease is that doctors love to incorporate, fill out prescriptions, and hand out hefty bills knowing full well you're not covered by insurance and, [having just been] approved by Social Security, you're also not covered by Medicare, because there is a twenty-four-month waiting period!! What the hell, I've been fighting Social Security since 1977, was finally approved in July of 1980—when 1982 rolls around I will have had lupus for seven years! Let's hope we have a cure by then!

I would *love* to go back to work as a floor broker on the Chicago Board Options Exchange and regain my vice president's title!!

We must remember that SLE is a personal, individual disease that includes *men* as well as women!!

Dr. Theodore Nadelson, chief of psychiatry, Boston Veterans' Administration Hospital, and clinical professor of psychiatry, Tufts University Medical School, says, "There may be many fantasies on the part of men who have been told that lupus is a disease predominantly of women. When the disease takes its toll, they also feel fatigued, and may believe they are losing their masculine sexuality. For some men this becomes too great a burden. They feel alienated, damaged, and emasculated. They also need a sturdy counselor-physician to guide them through many difficulties and to reassure them that their fatigue is not caused by changing sexuality, but by their immune system. I believe that one important issue with this disease, then, is that patients with it need support—support from the medical profession, support from their families, and support from one another. They need that until a remission occurs or a cure can be found. Such support, of course, assumes knowledgeable physicians—doctors who know about the disease and understand human despair and can respond to both these aspects in a human way. That is asking a lot, but this disease asks a lot of the sufferer as well."

Dr. Peter Schur, professor of medicine at Harvard University Medical School and director of lupus research at Brigham and Women's Hospital, stresses that there are a number of investigations going on right now regarding lupus in men as compared to lupus in women.

In particular, the group at Wellesley Hospital in Toronto, under the direction of Dr. Murray Urowitz, has done a great deal of research on male and female lupus patients. Dr. Schur has also conducted some clinical studies at Harvard University Medical School. In addition, Dr. Robert Lahita at Rockefeller University is conducting studies on sex hormones in both male and female lupus patients. Dr. Norman Talal's studies on the role of sex hormones in mice with lupus have been described in Chapter 4.

The mean age of onset of lupus in males is thirty-nine, according to a study by Dr. Urowitz.* This is slightly older than the average onset in females. However, onset in males occurs anywhere from fourteen to sixty-three years of age. The clinical manifestations in male and female lupus patients appear almost identical, although the Toronto study noted somewhat more pleuritis (lung inflammation) in males and less alopecia (baldness) and thrombocytopenia (reduction in the number of platelets) in males. The severity and mortality rate among males and females was the same in the Toronto study, although Dr. Schur's studies project a somewhat higher mortality in males.

It is clear that while lupus is far more prevalent among women, it can be equally devastating—perhaps even more so—to men experiencing it. It is to be hoped that the growing public awareness of lupus will benefit not only the many women affected by it, but also this often-ignored group of male lupus patients.

* M.H. Miller et al., "SLE in Males," *Medicine* 62: 327, 1982.

15

Lupus in Children

Living with lupus is never easy, regardless of one's age. But to me, children with lupus are like birds with broken wings. They miss the freedom to run and play in the bright sunshine, and they have to learn, painfully, to cope with a disease that greatly alters their lives.

In the past few years I have spoken to many children and teenagers afflicted with lupus; many have had great difficulty in adjusting to the disease. However, some are striving to function normally, and quite a few succeed. Some teenagers with lupus appear preoccupied with religion; some are depressed and withdrawn; some abandon their studies and their friends; and some refuse to rest or stay out of the sun, ignoring the advice of their physicians or parents. Still others, despite adverse changes in the laboratory tests, insist that they feel fine; they are determined not to take prescribed steroids, and thus avoid the moon face caused by the retention of fluids. One fourteen-year-old girl said: "I flush the cortisone pills in the toilet and then refill the bottle with aspirin tablets." Some parents have difficulty dealing with such situations without appearing overprotective and despotic, while others find themselves in a bind, especially with other siblings in the family. Sometimes the healthy children cannot understand why their brother or sister, who frequently looks well, gets all the attention. They fail to understand why they are scolded for having a C average in school, while the sibling with lupus may be praised for similar grades. Parents become especially worried if their healthy child begins to change in personality and behavior and emulates the brother or sister who has the disease.

According to Dr. Theodore Nadelson, chief of psychiatry at Boston Veterans' Administration Hospital and clinical professor of psychiatry at Tufts University Medical School: "The fact is, of course, that a young patient treated in a special way may miss being encouraged toward discipline and increased resolve. The parents' dilemma is that they may be straining the youngster beyond his or her capacity."

How can one help the young lupus patient to rebuild determination and strive for continued growth? How can one help the parents? Dr. Nadelson says:

"Any child has difficulty if he or she feels 'different' while growing up. To be the same as others is to be acceptable. Children who are perceived as different are often ostracized and ridiculed. This is the reason they all want to dress alike, eat the same foods, have the same likes, and so forth. If they don't, they risk being thought of as strange or 'weird.' The fact is that the disease does make them different, at times markedly. If it is not the lesions, then it is the fact that they cannot, for example, sunbathe like the rest of the kids. Developing adolescents are terribly concerned about their appearance. To be different means to risk being shut out from others in the group, and being shut out is tantamount, in the adolescent, to abandonment and even death. This disease almost certainly pushes them into a category of *not* belonging. Their frequent fatigue and the perspective of a long chronic illness adds to these sources of potential difficulty. Of course, parents may tend to overprotect the child with lupus, and that leads to the perception of inequities within the family. The effect on the other family members, of course, makes having the disease doubly hard. Much of the work has to do with the parents' determination to raise youngsters in a normal way, yet they recognize that in many ways the youngster is not normal. As the young person grows older, the question arises, should he or she marry? Will he or she be able to deal with the difficulties of marriage along with the difficulties of the disease? Parents need to be firm in their resolution to build within the youngsters the determination to help themselves. The young person must learn to deal with reality, and that includes the fact of lupus. The disease does add another burden to an adolescent already weighed down by the difficulties of growing up. The parents must acknowledge this, and at the same time help the youngster continue to develop as normally as possible.

"Sometimes a child gains certain distinctions so that he or she is regarded as special without having to *be* special, because of his or her disease. But most parents need the help of a knowledgeable physician to guide and advise them on the development of the child. The parents can gain a cognitive handle on the problem by consulting the physician on matters that might be difficult for them to see clearly. For example, the issue of sexuality is even more difficult for a child with lupus. Again, I focus on this area because it is important for the developing adolescent. It can be a particular problem for the teenaged lupus patient, who may feel deprived of the pleasures of normal interaction between the sexes. This can lead to artificial behavior—excessive promiscuity, for example. It can also go in the opposite direction, toward a kind of sexual retardation or inhibition. Parents should discuss this with their physician. If necessary, in the face of family inhibitions, doctors must promote such discussions by asking questions." Dr. Nadelson stresses that the Lupus Foundation of America (see Chapter 17) can continue to help arm the physician for such questions through literature emphasizing that the doctor must be not only the dispenser of medication, but also a counselor and supporter to the family in trouble. "I also wonder," Dr. Nadelson said, "and this is absolute conjecture, whether an adolescent female might feel more comfortable talking to a woman physician than she would to a man."

Depression can also be a problem in youngsters with lupus. According to Dr. Nadelson, "The way to prevent depression is to assemble helping, caring, yet firm and constant figures who will be supportive and, at the same time, encourage independence. Adolescents have quite a job to do in terms of maturation and development, and we can try to keep the process as normal as possible despite the burden of lupus. For some people, and this may sound strangely optimistic, just having the disease does not retard development; it may lead, instead, to greater strength for the individual. This is always an extremely exciting and refreshing thing to see."

Vicki Croke is such an exciting and inspiring young patient. I have known Vicki since she was a sophomore in high school, and she is now a graduate of the University of Massachusetts with a degree in journalism. For the past two years, Vicki has been employed by the *Boston Herald*. In her spare time, Vicki helps me with *Lupus News*.* Vicki is presently a patient of Dr. Yves Borel, who will present the clinical picture of lupus in children later in this chapter. Vicki wrote:

> I learned that I had lupus in the fall of 1971, just after my thirteenth birthday, and, oddly enough, just after receiving the Presidential Physical Fitness Award. At the time, my only symptom was a butterfly-shaped rash stretching across the bridge of my nose and onto my cheeks. Although I felt fine physically, emotionally I felt disabled by the restrictions my doctor put on my life-style.
>
> Adjusting to the disease was just impossible for me. I was only thirteen, and, while all my friends tried out for cheerleading, I sat under the bleachers and out of the sun. As my physical condition worsened I became more distraught. I became violently ill the winter of 1973, when I was fifteen years old.
>
> I had gaping mouth sores, aching swollen joints, fever, weight loss, irritated butterfly rash, an unrelenting fatigue, low white blood cell count, and inflammation of the membrane surrounding the lungs. For the first time I had to face my disease. I discovered that systemic lupus erythematosus is a powerful force to be reckoned with. I was too weak and too ill to refuse my medication—prednisone. From my sparse bits of information I viewed it with vague dread, knowing that the dangers of prolonged intake of massive doses are shocking.
>
> And the side effects I experienced lived up to my expectations. I gained weight; I became a "moon face" due to retention of fluids; I suffered high blood pressure, a hip disorder, and mysterious knee pains. I also recorded dry skin and stretch marks. I stopped growing in height and had dizzy spells, nausea, and other day-to-day annoyances.
>
> The disease had chased me into the shadows, and now, too weak to fight back, I was given a medication that distorted my face and wiped away much of my identity. Although I knew that this disfigurement was only temporary, the experience of seeing someone else in the mirror left me

---

* *Lupus News*, the national newspaper of the Lupus Foundation of America, has a circulation of over 50,000. Editor, Henrietta Aladjem.

devastated. When I got out of the hospital, I did not attend school, but had tutors. I did not allow my friends to visit, and I refused to leave the house.

I went out once on the encouragement of a friend over the phone. I went to see a school production of *Camelot*—I met all my friends in the balcony, and not one of them recognized me. I went home with a spirit even more changed than my face.

Dependence on medical caretakers and parents and a monitored life-style all set the regression in motion.

I had read that the normal development of children includes a movement from passivity to activity, from dependence to independence, from ambiguous sexual identity to a definite one, and from total involvement with self to concern for others as well. Whatever progress I had made with these steps not only stopped but reversed itself.

I hid from the world inside my home. I was passive, dependent, sexually ambiguous, and self-centered. I was content with the situation for a few months, happily absorbing the unconditional, doting love of my parents. My mother took a leave of absence from work and would ride buses on freezing February days to spend every one of my hospital days beside me. My father would arrive late, grimy and exhausted from a full day's labor as a truck driver. They would drive home together in the chilled darkness, long after visiting hours were over. Their devotion did not end when I returned home from the hospital.

I left all decisions up to my family. My sister, then working at Filene's, bought all my clothes and brought them home to me. I would cook, but someone had to tell me what to make, and if I disagreed with someone, I just gave in, which was not at all like myself.

When the few friends I hadn't scared away called, their talk of "the boys" was alien to me. I just felt too unattractive to think of myself as a sexual being. I saw myself more as some sort of eunuch.

Finally, I was totally self-centered. I spent much of my day alone in the house. I was my only companion, and rumination was my only activity.

I did very well with my school work; it was a life preserver to hang onto and eventually a base to build on. But I was very depressed. I was dependent, fragile, and passive. I felt that for some reason God chose to punish me, and there was nothing I could do about it.

At some point, I don't know when and I don't know why, the depression focused—I was too tired of being sick, too tired of being fat, too tired of being passive, dependent, friendless, and self-centered. I suddenly realized that I was a straight-A student. I went on a diet, my medication was reduced gradually, and I even began to see a few friends on a regular basis.

It is here that for the second time in my life, there was a movement from passivity to activity; the other steps of the emotional progression did not occur so rapidly, however. I built up my courage and returned to school in the fall of 1974. During the next two years my disease went into remission, my dependence shifted from parents to friends to approaching independence, my sexual identity became more definite as I began to mingle with "the boys," and as my concern for others grew, my unhealthy involvement with self withered.

There is a symbiosis between mind and body. And the growth of my social life reinforced, and was reinforced by, my rapidly improving health. I was voted class wit, I graduated with honors, with friends, and in remission.

I think that a vital part of a chronically ill patient's well-being is the doctor-patient relationship. My relationship with my doctor was a nasty one. She was cold, bullying, and at times downright sadistic. She once gave me an injection in my upper lip without a painkiller, and without a warning about the pain. To this day I shudder when I think of that clinic visit.

I viewed my doctor as the personification of the disease, and therefore with hatred. She kept my family in the dark about aspects of the disease, the side effects of some of the drugs, and even once about the type of surgery about to be performed on me! Yet we knew of few doctors treating lupus at the time, and scientifically, she was one of the best.

I spent my clinic visits telling her she just couldn't understand what it was like to have lupus. We might have spent even more visits this way, but she died in the fall of 1974. After her death I learned that she had been suffering from lupus herself!

We could have shared a knowledge of a common suf-

if only she had told me. But instead, at age sixteen, I was left with the enigma of a doctor, a healer, too uptight about the disease she was treating me for to tell me that she had it also. She denied the disease, went out in the sun, exerted herself, and died very young. Perhaps I, as a lupus patient, represented the disease she could not control as a sufferer, or as a physician, as much as she personified lupus to me. But this is just one of the many questions I have that will remain unanswered.

My current physician is known as a leader in the field of immunological research; his candor, warmth, and emotional support, however, are as important to me as his scientific reputation. He has taught me to relax with lupus, and so my good health continued.

I am now at ease with lupus. It is part of me. I do not ignore that, but it does not define who I am. I am not shattered by aching joints, fevers, or fatigue (which all exist when the disease is in remission), and I am not afraid to tell people about it. I face a sunny future—umbrella in hand, of course.

Lisa Chin, a bright and sensitive eleven-year-old girl, describes how it feels to be her age and strive to function normally.

You asked me how does it feel to be eleven and have lupus. I am grumpy and in pain and I don't want to admit it. One can ask me a simple question and I'll burst into tears for no reason. I am bedridden one day and I feel better the next. When I am too tired to do something, I wonder, is this feeling really true or am I just using lupus as an excuse not to do my homework? I want to be treated like a normal girl, but I also have to be dealt with depending on how I feel that day. I need understanding! I need somebody willing to hear out my problems. My only support system is my three-year-old brother Mike. He listens when I tell him how tired and sick I feel and he gives me the kisses and hugs I need that everyone else says I am "too old for." I would like a friend or someone to give me support, but my parents always say, "Nobody wants to listen to a girl who complains all the time." Sometimes, if I feel rotten, I think of how easy it would be "to get it over with." I also say, "Why should I try to be on top of the class? I could be dead tomorrow!"

I quickly put these thoughts aside and say to myself, "Why kill yourself? If you're dead when they find a cure how would Mom and Dad feel? You're dead so it doesn't matter, but Mom and Dad would be pretty upset.

"Be at the top of the class! If you drop dead tomorrow you'll die a smart kid who didn't give up." For someone who's got nothing to live for, I've got a lot of reasons to keep living; I just have to take each day as it comes.

Dr. Raquel Hicks of the John A. Burns School of Medicine in Honolulu, Hawaii, wrote the following passage entitled, "Butterflies, Sunshine and Rainbows, or, Caring for Children with Lupus in Hawaii." Dr. Hicks is director of the Pediatric Arthritis Center of Hawaii, and associate professor of pediatrics and medicine.

"Hawaii is considered by many one of the most beautiful spots in the world. It has been praised by poets and song composers because of its natural beauty and perfect harmony of nature, as sun, sea, and beautiful living things of many colors and shapes display themselves before the eyes of the incredulous visitor. Perfect weather all year round, perfumed trade winds, waterfalls, warm waters, rainbows, and white sand offer a pleasant environment to both *malahini* (newcomer) and *kamaaina* (longtime resident) alike.

"But the real beauty of Hawaii resides in its people, of many lands, and the rich mixture of colors and temperaments that give Hawaiians that special beauty of body and spirit. A friendly smile on a morning jog, a wave of the hand from a stranger, a basket of fruit recently picked, or a lei of flowers—destiny brought me to Paradise fourteen years ago. I am a real lover of these islands.

"Practicing as a pediatric rheumatologist for this length of time has allowed me to see my children grow, get well, get married and have their own children, move away, at times share with their family in their sorrow when systemic lupus gets ahead of our state-of-the-art therapy. However, my life has been blessed, for I have met many wonderful people that have made my life richer: Lynn, Ken, Sibyl, Heather, Lorene, Wendy, Natalie, Sharin, Delia, Emma-Jean, Margaret, Joanne, Lovey, and others. The diagnosis of lupus. The fear. The incredible notion that maybe from now on, a carefree life-style would be replaced by blood tests, doctors' visits, and avoidance of sun exposure. The blame. The acceptance. Christmas gifts mixed with lab slips. A new dress with a blood spot. A hospital admission to intensive care. Is it infection? Is it a flareup? Fear. Why me, Doctor Hicks? Friends. Always there.

"Graduation, flower leis, so high it's hard to see. I have to hold my tears back. These special children mean so much to me. Some move, some stay. But all remembered.

"Throughout the years, experience has taught me that generalizations don't work, and that demands only set off oppositional behaviors in adolescents and children. This is true in my own household, as my own kids, now sixteen and thirteen, actually have inadvertently slipped into the feared teenage years with great maturity and wisdom. Compromising is the name of the game.

"My Hawaiian patients, restricted from the sun, are allowed to swim in the evening. Tennis players can go about their game on a reduced training schedule or as the condition permits. Long sleeves, cotton or gauze white blouses, colorful visors, luuhulu hats, and a thick layer of sunscreen are recommended. The beach is as beautiful in the evening, and the water is warmer. A family picnic under the palm trees, watching a spectacular sunset, seems attractive enough. These allowances have a price: moderation, and the promise to pace, and rest. Children soon find out that overdoing causes flareups. But children they are, and they must experiment as they go about their business.

"Because of the multicultural background of our population, we must deal with a variety of cultural beliefs in our families. We have found out that we must keep our own personal education at a high level so we can discuss these matters intelligently—Chinese herbal remedies, Shiatsu massage, and traditional Hawaiian culture (no'oponopono) are some of the beliefs we must learn to deal with. Through understanding and education, and the assistance of linguists and visual aids, we have been successful in incorporating our own beliefs into these rich ancient cultures.

"One major complaint is the loss of hair experienced by some as a result of disease or medication. Those long, black, beautiful tresses. It will come back! Much thicker, much healthier. We make a joke about it. Do you think I might get blonde hair? The laughter stops the worry at least temporarily. Waiting is hard. I know. How about short hair for a while? It's cooler, and *very* becoming. Few wear a wig, since it is too hot. Most wear a cap. Flowers in the hair are so becoming, and great to conceal bald spots, I'm told.

" 'Give me attitude,' my outspoken dear friend Jerry Jacobs said at a local meeting. I agree. Children must face society and its pressures. They must deal with unkind comments, teasing, mockery, curiosity, from peers and well-meaning family members. We try to emphasize a self-reliant attitude. No lies, kids. But usually complicated explanations are not well understood by children. They may say something like, 'I'm having trouble with my hair. The doctor says I have problems with my skin,' or, 'I have a sun allergy.' They are encouraged to share as much as they feel comfortable with.

"Incorporating the child as a member of the treatment team sounds like a good idea. How to do it is another story. I recently became convinced that we are missing the boat if we don't take a [medical] history from the child, too. A precocious two-year-old girl, Jennifer, proved this to me. Jennifer had developed Kawasaki syndrome [a disease affecting the lymph nodes] with arthritis. When her mother mentioned that she was limping, but that the source of the limp was unclear, Jennifer interrupted, saying, 'My knee hurts, Mommie.' She knew best. In my program, the Pediatric Arthritis Center of Hawaii, we have attempted to face this problem by developing educational material made especially for children. The 'For You' series now includes pamphlets: 'For You, a Child with Juvenile Rheumatoid Arthritis'; 'For You, a Teenager with Lupus.' We are working on pamphlets for rheumatic fever and Kawasaki syndrome, common disorders in the Islands. We are now working on translating these pamphlets into the various languages spoken in the Islands and evaluating the impact of this material in our population of children.

"Building up confidence and ego strength has been a full-time job for the parents and my team. We emphasize what they *can* do, not what they can't do. If you're a competitive surfer, a marathoner, find out what *else* you like. Strengthen your legs. Swim laps in an indoor pool. Maybe some day! In the meantime, you may have to jog, not run, or walk, and not jog. It all depends.

"But at times, a carefree life-style of outdoor activities is more important than anything else, and acceptance is poor. The surfer, the marathoner, the tennis player, all attempt 'going back to the way it was,' with painful learning experiences. Moderation is the name of the game. My kids have seen me grow, too, from the busy thirties to the active forties. Yes, learning goes both ways. Yes, it's okay to worry."

Dr. Yves Borel is an associate professor of pediatrics, Harvard University Medical School, and director of rheumatology services, Children's Medical Center. He is currently taking care of about forty young persons with lupus. According to Dr. Borel, the number of young patients with lupus at Children's Medical Center has doubled in the past four or five years. The majority of these children, Dr. Borel says, are doing relatively well.

Dr. Borel describes briefly the onset, the clinical manifestations, and the management of SLE in children.

THE AGE OF ONSET

Systemic lupus erythematosus is the second most common connective tissue disease in children, after juvenile rheumatoid arthritis, but preceding dermatomyositis or scleroderma. The age of onset varies, but generally falls between four and eighteen years. Before four years of age lupus is extremely rare. A few reports are known of mothers with active systemic lupus whose babies had a facial rash and some of the serological manifestations of systemic lupus erythematosus. This represents a passive transfer of antibodies from the mother to the fetus, and as a rule both the clinical and serological manifestations spontaneously disappear after a few months. Systemic lupus is not genetically transmitted in a classical dominant Mendelian way. Most children of mothers with lupus are healthy, although in some children an increase occurs in the incidence of heart block. Both boys and girls can have lupus, but in children, as in adults, lupus overwhelmingly predominates in girls. The ratio of lupus in females to males varies from 4:1 to 9:1, depending on the clinical center. The peak incidence of lupus among youngsters is at adolescence, where girls are most often affected. This supports the view that female hormones do play a role in accelerating or worsening the disease, in contrast to male hormones, which have the opposite effect. Thus, women are known to form greater amounts of antibodies than males, and to be more prone to autoimmune diseases.

THE MODE OF ONSET
AND THE CLINICAL MANIFESTATIONS

How does lupus manifest itself in children? Is lupus different in children than in adults? The answer is that the symptoms are the same in children and adults in the majority of cases (60–90 percent), but a few clinical manifestations are unique to children. In the vast majority of cases the mode of onset is the classical facial rash, fever, and arthralgia. It may start with, for instance, low-grade fever and fatigue, or arthralgia and proteinuria (protein in the urine), or a butterfly facial rash in a girl with a positive antinuclear antibody test. But many girls who have facial rashes and even a low titer of antinuclear antibody do not have lupus. Uncommon symptoms of onset are seizures, abdominal pain, and bleeding from the gastrointestinal tract, or purpura (the escape of blood from the capillaries into the skin or mucous membranes). Hemolytic anemia may also be the first symptom of lupus. One mode of onset unique to children is juvenile rheumatoid arthritis associated with enlargement of the spleen, glandular disease, and high titers of antinuclear antibody. Despite these abnormal autoimmune markers, this form of the disease has a good prognosis. Thus, lupus in its atypical mode of onset could affect, initially, the kidney, the central nervous system, the blood, or exclusively the joints. For example, a child may have a single epileptic seizure at age four, and ten years later develop lupus. Alternatively, kidney inflammation with persistent unexplained proteinuria may be the first symptom of the disease. Because lupus can be present in many different forms, sick children with possible SLE must be referred to an academic medical center equipped to make the diagnosis.

The criteria for the diagnosis have been recently updated to include antibody to native DNA and anti-sm antibody, which are typically characteristic of the disease. As with the diagnosis of lupus in adults, one needs four criteria to make the diagnosis in children, which may include either clinical manifestations or serological findings. The natural course of the disease varies from one child to another, and for each patient the course is unique. Fortunately, most children get better spontaneously. A few adolescents have severe life-threatening disease, whereas others will continue to have relapses and remissions all their lives. What dictates the severity of the disease is the extent of organ involvement. Often, the most severe disease occurs in black girls, although the incidence of the disease is also higher in blacks in general. Three broad manifestations of the disease have a poor prognosis: lupus nephritis (kidney involvement), CNS involvement, and persistent systemic manifestations. While each of these might be a cause of death, none of them in itself is a cause for despair, because they can be successfully treated or even get better on their own. The prognosis of the disease has improved considerably and continues to improve each year. Five years after the diagnosis, 95 percent of all children with lupus are alive.

MANAGEMENT OF THE DISEASE

For the young adult, the disease arrives at a time when many other problems of adolescence have to be faced and solved. The child is experiencing difficulties with personal identity, independence, and sexual awareness, to mention just a few of the problems facing teenagers. His or her treatment should reflect an understanding of these issues.

How the young adult deals with his or her illness varies enormously from one teenager to another. The response is also dependent on the seriousness of the illness. Parents should encourage their sick child to lead a normal life, to attend school, and to participate in social and physical activities to the fullest extent possible. Children are much more direct and spontaneous than adults. In some instances, to be sick will depress them, but in others it will help motivate them. Most young adults with lupus are intelligent and perceptive and have an inborn capacity to adjust to what is still an unknown and confusing illness.

The treatment is dictated both by the clinical manifestations and the severity of the disease. For example, if the main symptoms are skin rash and arthralgia, aspirin and/or Plaquenil is the treatment of choice. But if the symptoms include severe Coombes-positive hemolytic anemia or purpura, the treatment of choice is prednisone. One should avoid giving steroids unless the disease cannot be controlled without them. The three stages of the treatment are aspirin and Plaquenil; steroids; and immunosuppressive drugs or treatment (Imuran, Cytoxan, and/or plasmapheresis). Almost all children with lupus, like adults with active systemic disease, are on steroids. In addition to the well-known side effects of steroids, including osteoporosis, pathologic fractures, and cataracts, the moon faces and the weight gain caused by steroids may be difficult to accept for a youngster concerned with his or her personal appearance. Occasionally, patients refuse to take prednisone. One should taper the steroids as soon as possible and, where possible, give them on alternate days to permit normal growth. However, other immunosuppressive drugs are available. For example, Imuran is a steroid-sparing drug that is very effective in some cases with systemic manifestations. By contrast, Cytoxan appears to be the drug of choice in central nervous system or steroid-resistant renal lupus.

A LOOK AT THE FUTURE

Although the cause of the disease is still unknown, medical specialists appear to agree that lupus represents a disorder of immunoregulation. Tissue damage is caused by immune complexes, mainly to nucleic acid antigens. One of the main goals of future therapy is the specific suppression of antibody to DNA, because this will provide an antigen-specific therapy for the disease instead of the nonspecific suppression produced by steroids or other immunosuppressive drugs. This idea has been supported by the finding that immunologic tolerance to DNA antigens can be induced not only in experimental animals *in vivo* (in living tissue), but also in human peripheral blood lymphocytes from SLE patients *in vitro* (in glass, as in a test tube). In addition, a new method was recently developed to link fragments of DNA to a protein carrier. This is particularly significant because fragments of DNA have the antibody-combining site made by SLE patients. In addition, the specificity of the family of antibodies made by lupus patients is apparently more restricted than originally thought. They may recognize common structures present on different antigens. Since this common antigenic determinant is present in DNA fragments, it is conceivable that when linked to appropriate self molecules, such as human gamma globulin, they may provide a powerful substance that specifically suppresses the formation of unwanted antibody. In any event, this new approach will permit a test of the hypothesis that autoimmunity can be treated by the creation of specific immunologic tolerance.

CONCLUSION

Dr. Malcolm Rogers, a psychiatrist at Brigham and Women's Hospital in Boston, commented: "The special quality of the children and adolescents with lupus that shines through is their resiliency. Despite the psychological trauma created by the disease and the interruptions in their activities, kids continue to grow and develop compensatory strengths. Even when she was in her most depressed state, Vicki Croke was studying hard and would rebuild, in time, her self-esteem around that. It is this resiliency that allows so many of these children to continue to lead normal lives in spite of lupus."

16

Lupus and the Workplace: The Special Problems of Social Security Disability and Job Discrimination

Lupus patients have great difficulty obtaining Social Security Disability. They have problems because neither judges nor Social Security investigators tend to be familiar with the disease, and they lack guidelines that would help determine whether the patient can work. And many patients find it difficult to obtain employment or keep a job because of their medical condition and the lack of understanding of the ups and downs of this illness.

Monica B. Gilliam of Detroit wrote this letter to the Social Security Administration (SSA):

> Please direct your attention to the fact that since 1977 my disease has progressed, in spite of continuous treatment, at a somewhat rapid rate. Initially there were multiple arthralgias and decreased pulmonary function. Subsequent flares have caused further damage, consequently creating problems in terms of activities of daily living. Medical records confirm that I was hospitalized several times for exacerbations of SLE.

My rheumatologist considered adding antimalarial drugs to my present course of therapy with the hope of halting the progression of the disease. However such drugs are contraindicated. . . . I have extensive retinal damage.

It is a known fact among SLE patients that regardless of laboratory findings, most of the time we feel quite sick, lack energy, have joint and muscle pains, and experience great difficulty performing our duties, even simple personal care. These symptoms are intermittent and vary from day to day, sometimes even during the course of the same day. Only someone who sees me frequently can testify about my performance.

The medications I must take for control of symptoms cause drowsiness and lethargy. As a nurse, I must be alert and able to perform whenever my patients need my services. Otherwise I become a danger to the patients and increase the risk of legal liability on my part and that of the hospital for which I work.

My job also requires my driving to patients' homes at times to render nursing care and supervise others. At present I am unable to drive myself for my therapy at the Rehabilitation Institute three times per week. Stair climbing is also difficult—how can I serve these patients?

I have not asked to be placed on medical disability for an indefinite period. I could not live with that thought. My strength of will makes me believe that I will experience a remission. However, it is unlikely that a remission will be attained if I am forced to return to my job while I am still impaired. It is my perception that SSA is forcing me to work, without regard for my pains and other symptoms. I am simply requesting my pro-rated benefits until my health improves.

There are times when I am unable to hold a pen due to painful fingers and wrist, even when swelling is minimal. It is evident there are contractures of my hand. I need assistance getting dressed at times—even your doctors had to assist me when they performed the exams you demanded. You mentioned that according to my X rays there's lack of joint pathology. Please be informed that unlike arthritis, SLE joint pains and weakness seem to be caused mainly by affected tendons, not bone degeneration.

I have cooperated and submitted to rather uncomfortable

examinations, on two occasions, by doctors of your choice. The diagnosis has been confirmed. The degree of my symptoms varies. Presently I am very uncomfortable sitting, needless to mention walking, due to skin eruption.

Rejecting by SSA has aggravated my situational depression, because I (and persons who know me well) know that I love my work; therein lies my strength. I have put much effort into my career, and have written recognition to show. As soon as I am able, you will not need to force me to return. In 1978 I returned to work full-time under my own direction, not my doctors'. Even though I was not well, I was better and wanted to work. I still want to try, but I am having greater difficulty doing so at this time. Furthermore my doctors advise much rest—I am told that rest is probably the most important therapy. You seem to be telling me to go against my physicians' advice.

Perhaps you may need to revise your protocol with assistance from systemic lupus erythematosus sufferers who can give you firsthand information about a disease which, most experts in the field agree, is unpredictable, puzzling, and incurable—a disease that requires much further research.

Another lupus patient who was denied disability in New Jersey wrote:

In a statement received from the SSI, they said my joint pain will subside and I will be able to resume gainful employment within a year. This statement is ridiculous. At eight months, I still suffer from joint pain in the fingers, wrists, elbows, shoulders, knees, and ankles. If I totally rest, the pain is controllable with twelve aspirin a day, prednisone (steroids), and anti-malarial drugs; but any type of physical activity brings the pain back. Minimal typing is an excruciating experience.

In addition, the Board has not taken into account the numerous other involvements I suffer from. These include weakness; fatigue; dizziness; spasms of the small blood vessels in the fingertips and toes following slight exposure to cold or emotional stimulation, which decrease the blood supply and cause blanching of the skin and considerable pain in the fingertips and feet; extreme sensitivity to ultraviolet radiation including sunlight, fluorescent light, and Xerox machines (upon being subjected for brief periods of ten to fifteen minutes, the disease exacerbates, immediately causing dizziness, weakness, painful neuropathy, and mood changes; longer exposure leads to a systemic flare—being allergic to PABA, which is in sunscreens, and since the sunscreens without PABA do not work to protect me, this particular involvement of the disease is extremely difficult); shortness of breath; kidney pain; burning with urination; painful neuropathy in feet, hands, face, center of spine at waist, and top of spine at neck; difficulty walking with heaviness in legs; wild mood swings; forgetfulness and excitability; difficulty with concentration; sensitivity to heat; exacerbation of disease upon encountering stress.

All the aforementioned involvements are well-documented problems encountered by lupus patients. I am one of those patients who has experienced all of them.

I truly believe that whoever made the decision on my behalf and disallowed my claim had absolutely NO KNOWLEDGE OF THE DISEASE SYSTEMIC LUPUS ERYTHEMATOSUS. To be disabled by lupus has been heartbreaking; to have the federal government deny me the security I have worked for and paid to have, is a travesty of justice.

About six years ago, I went to court with a lupus patient in Rhode Island. After we testified she was granted Social Security Disability. Two years later, the woman had to be hospitalized with a heart condition, and shortly after, she was taken off Social Security Disability. I went to court with her again, this time in Boston, and despite our pleading, the judge ruled that she was in remission and therefore could work. This decision defied all logic. I went with the patient to see her doctor, a well-known clinician in Boston, and asked him to write a letter to explain her condition to the judge. This is what the doctor wrote:

Mrs. Merry Lorenz has been under my care for systemic lupus erythematosus since March 1975. She has had a stormy course over the subsequent years, but fortunately her disease has been better controlled recently. She presented with severe autoimmune-hemolytic anemia, which required high doses of corticosteroids. Subsequently, she had a severe multisystem flare with severe renal disease, hypertension, hepatitis, arthritis, and pleurisy with some myocardial involvement. There was also central nervous system involvement, which also gradually cleared on therapy.

In 1979, she suffered an acute myocardial infarction and was hospitalized at the Massachusetts General Hospital. She recovered uneventfully from this but continued to have difficulty controlling hypertension in spite of multiple antihypertensive medications, approximately four medications at a time. Over the past few months, a new combination of medications has resulted in better control of her hypertension, and her systemic lupus appears to be quiescent.

There is no question that Merry's systemic lupus, although quiescent at the present time, has not been cured, and she will always have a tendency to have flares if various exogenous stresses or other unknown factors come to pass that can aggravate the disease. Although the scientific data on behalf of rest therapy for systemic lupus is incomplete, there is a strong feeling among authorities that rest is a very important aspect of the management of this disease. This is most forcefully expressed in the monograph *Systemic Lupus Erythematosus* by Marian W. Ropes, published by Harvard University Press in 1976, in which she strongly encourages a strict rest program in order to allow the patient to maintain maximum resistence to the resurgence of the disease activity. In addition, lupus patients are known to be susceptible to infection, and it is important for patients with a background of systemic lupus to minimize their contacts with sources of infection in individuals outside their home. Because of the seriousness of the systemic lupus Mrs. Lorenz has experienced in the past, her management must be continued to be taken very seriously. Because of the presence of cardiac disease, although not active at the present time, any failure of control of her hypertension would be detrimental as well. Both from the point of view of control of her hypertension and in particular in order to maintain her disease in its current quiescent state, I feel it is vital that she have limited work scheduled to essential tasks in the care of her home and family, and that she not work outside of her home. As her physician and rheumatologist, I can certainly not take the responsibility to advise her to return to work at this time. I believe if she attempted to carry out full-time work that this could have a deleterious effect on the course of her disease, which has been life-threatening in the past.

Thank you for consideration of this matter.

This letter was disregarded by the Social Security office, and the patient is still appealing her case.

I asked Elizabeth Jameson, an attorney on the board of directors of the Lupus Foundation of America, to explain how our Social Security Administration works. Attorney Jameson wrote:

"The federal government, via the Social Security Administration, administers two separate programs for work. One program is the Social Security Disability Program (SSD). This program provides monthly benefits to disabled workers who have established a considerable work history in Social Security-covered employment. Because women often have periods when they have been out of the paid work force, many lupus patients are not able to meet this requirement. Those who are ineligible for SSD because they do not meet the work requirement may be eligible to receive benefits under the Supplemental Security Income (SSI) program. SSI eligibility is based on the applicant's minimal income and resources, and on whether he or she meets the age or disability requirements. It is not dependent on an employment history covered by Social Security.

"In order to qualify for cash benefits under either of these programs, a person must be considered legally 'disabled.' Hundreds of persons who have been diagnosed as having lupus, or who suffer from an as yet undiagnosed disease, are found to be ineligible for benefits on the basis that they do not meet the necessary definition of 'disabled' under the terms of the two programs.

"The word *disability* is a legal term, and is defined as the inability to engage in substantial gainful work because of a physical or mental impairment that has lasted or is expected to last for at least twelve months, or that can be expected to result in death. Generally, an individual who cannot perform ordinary or simple tasks satisfactorily is considered unable to engage in substantial gainful employment. Before being entitled to benefits, those who are unable to engage in 'substantial gainful employment' must establish that their inability to work arises from a 'severe impairment.' Under the Social Security Administration guidelines, a specific category of lupus patients is automatically considered 'severely impaired.' Those with lupus who have a positive LE preparation of biopsy or a positive ANA test, and who suffer from frequent exacerbations involving renal, cardiac, pulmonary, or gastrointestinal or central nervous system involvement, are considered to be 'severely impaired' for purposes of these programs. Such patients are therefore automatically entitled to benefits.

"Yet as many as 50 percent of lupus patients have negative LE preparations, and up to 10 percent of lupus patients have negative ANA test results. Those patients who have negative test results, along with those individuals who are awaiting diagnosis, may be considered 'severely impaired,' and therefore entitled to disability benefits, if the disease process imposes functional limitations on the individual's ability to engage in work-related activities. Yet the process of establishing disability without the positive test results is extremely difficult.

"Congress has structured these two programs so that those who claim to be too ill to work must have the burden of proving that they are eligible for benefits. While the claimant is entitled to present evidence of disability, the disease of lupus is characterized by various factors that are *not* currently recognized by the Social Security Administration. As described in previous chapters, many persons with lupus suffer from extreme fatigue. Others suffer from chronic pain. The Social Security Administration does not consider the existence of pain or fatigue and the effect debilitating pain and fatigue has on a person's ability to perform substantial gainful activity. Nor does the administration consider the combined effects of multiple nonsevere impairments. Most importantly, lupus is a disease characterized both by periods of acute illness and periods of remission. Test results are often confusing, and accurate diagnosis can take years. Current Social Security regulations are simply not responsive to the needs of thousands of individuals who suffer from lupus and who are too ill to work, but who do not have the necessary test results mandated by the regulations.

"On an optimistic note, many organizations have worked hard over the years to reform the disability programs so that all individuals too ill to work are able to survive economically in our society. In the past few years, Social Security Administration policies, in which hundreds of thousands of disabled individuals have been inappropriately terminated from the disability roles, have constituted a national scandal. The Social Security Administration's callous and inhumane disregard for those in our society who are too ill to work, and its refusal to assist these individuals in maintaining a subsistence level of existence, have resulted in the pain, suffering, and, in some instances, death of hundreds of thousands of disabled Americans. Organizations such as the Lupus Foundation of America have been working hard to reform our government programs and make them more responsive to the needs of their members.

"The United States Congress is currently considering passing major Social Security reform legislation that will address at least some of the major inequities in the administration of the Social Security Disability program. In the meantime, those with lupus who need economic assistance because of their inability to work should seek expert legal advice before taking on the long, hard road to obtaining disability benefits."

Deborah Thomson, an attorney on the board of directors of the Lupus Foundation of America, Massachusetts Chapter, wrote:

"Although lupus patients may have difficulty in obtaining Social Security Disability benefits, it is important to note that many patients win benefits during the appeal process. The Social Security Administration has an internal administrative process by which claimants who are initially denied in their claim for disability benefits can challenge that determination. The appeal process consists of five steps, beginning with the initial denial and culminating in a federal district court review of that denial. The crucial point in the appeal process for most claimants is step number three, the administrative hearing. Most reversals on claims occur at this level, and any further review is primarily based on the evidence submitted at the hearing.

"While it may seem clear to a claimant that he or she cannot work due to illness, this fact must be established in very specific ways before Social Security will grant a claimant benefits. In addition to requiring specific medical evidence, the Social Security regulations require a detailed analysis of a person's vocational skills and limitations. Because of the precise nature of the evidence required, it is essential that a claimant have the assistance of an advocate familiar with the appeals process. The advocate can ensure that the best possible evidentiary record is established, and that the patient testifies about those facets of his or her illness that clearly establish his or her disability.

"Although the cost of hiring an attorney may seem prohibitive, most attorneys are willing to take their fee out of any lump sum retroactive benefit award received by the claimant. If a patient is seeking SSI benefits, he or she can usually obtain free representation at a local legal services office. Depending on a claimant's work history, he or she may have great difficulty in reopening a Social Security claim once an adverse decision has been rendered. Thus it is very important to present as strong a case as possible on the first try.

"For many lupus patients the obtaining of Social Security Disability benefits is an exercise in frustration. The process is long (the appeals procedure can take years), seemingly irrational, and related less to one's actual health than to bureaucratic regulations. Yet those who are willing to fight stand a good chance of obtaining benefits on appeal. Only by fighting will sufferers of this elusive disease with its strange symptoms make our government aware that lupus is a serious and disabling illness within the meaning of the Social Security law and regulations."

For those lupus patients who do not seek or obtain disability benefits, the workplace poses special problems. Attorney Elizabeth Jameson further wrote:

"Many people who have chronic diseases are willing and able to continue in their present employment despite their medical condition. There is no typical lupus profile; some people go into remission for years at a time, while others only suffer from fatigue or pain on a periodic basis. The key legal question for those who want to work is whether employers can discriminate against those who suffer from major health problems.

"Examples of some of the legal problems that arise in the employment context are typified in the situation of a Cincinnati, Ohio, schoolteacher who was diagnosed as having lupus in 1982. She wished to continue teaching her fifth-grade class, but, due to her high degree of sun sensitivity, was no longer able to take the children outside for the noon recess. While she was able to perform satisfactorily the remainder of her teaching duties, she was terminated by her school district. A lab technician in San Jose, California, was no longer able to engage in heavy lifting after her diagnosis of lupus. In addition, she suffered from bouts of fatigue, requiring her to take occasional rest periods in the middle of the day. In all other respects, she was able to carry out satisfactorily her duties. She, too, was terminated from her job. Others with lupus complain of being turned down for promotions for which they were qualified, and others did not receive their pay increases. Many state that they were turned down for jobs when the employer discovered that the applicant had lupus.

"In the past ten years, a dramatic civil rights movement, aimed at the rights of the disabled in the workplace, resulted in the passage of major federal and state legislation.

"In 1973, Congress passed landmark legislation that guaranteed the rights of disabled Americans. This legislation, known as Title V of the Rehabilitation Act of 1973 (29 U.S.C. 701 *et seq.*), states that agencies of the federal government, federal aid recipients, and businesses receiving federal monies cannot discriminate against an individual because of a mental or physical handicap. Section 504 of the Rehabilitation Act is the broadest piece of federal legislation enacted to secure the rights of disabled persons.

"Lupus patients are entitled to the protections of this legislation if they fit one of the following definitions of the term *handicapped person*:

"(1) someone who has a physical or mental disability that substantially impairs or restricts one or more of such major life activities as walking, seeing, hearing, speaking, working, or learning;

"(2) someone who has a record of such a handicap, even though the person has recovered, is in remission, or has been misclassified as having a handicap, *or*

"(3) someone who is regarded as having handicaps, even though that handicap does not substantially limit the person's ability to function, or someone who does not have a handicap at all, but who is treated as if he or she had a substantially limiting handicap.

"Federal regulations state that handicapping conditions include, *but are not limited to:* alcoholism;* cancer; cerebral palsy; deafness

---

* The U.S. Attorney General has ruled that alcoholism and drug addiction are physical or mental impairments that are handicapping conditions if they limit one or more of life's major activities.

or hearing impairment; diabetes; drug addiction;* epilepsy; heart disease; mental or emotional illness; mental retardation; multiple sclerosis; muscular dystrophy; orthopedic, speech, or visual impairment; and perceptual handicaps such as dyslexia, minimal brain dysfunction, and developmental aphasia.

"The statutory definition of handicap encompasses the vast majority of lupus patients. A substantial percentage of lupus patients suffer from severe impairment of major life activities and are clearly covered under this legislation. Arguably, patients who currently suffer from lung, kidney, or heart involvement are automatically covered under this legislation.

"Individuals who once suffered from physical impairment due to lupus but who are currently in remission, and those individuals who have a history of lupus, are also covered under this legislation. In addition, the legislation is sufficiently broad to include in the definition of handicap those patients who suffer from such ailments as skin lesions or rashes and are not limited in their physical ability to function, but who are treated by others as if they did suffer from a limiting handicap. A belief on the part of others that a person has a disability, whether it is so or not, is recognized as a handicap under federal regulations.

"As a disabled job applicant or employee, lupus patients have the same rights and benefits as nonhandicapped applicants and employees. The lupus patient's ability, training, and experience must be considered. The disability must *not* be considered—unless it keeps the patient from doing the job adequately.

"An employer receiving federal assistance may not discriminate against qualified lupus patients in:

- recruitment, advertising, or processing of applications for employment

- physical examination; an applicant cannot be required to take a physical examination before a job is offered; the job applicant may be required to take a physical examination after the job is offered if the examination is required of other applicants

- hiring, promotion or demotion, transfer, layoff, or rehiring

- job assignments or career ladders
- leaves of absences, sick leave, training programs. and other fringe benefits.

"Once hired, an employer is required to take *reasonable steps to accommodate the lupus patient* unless it would cause the employer undue hardship. That may mean supplying, for example:

- adequate work space and access to it if the lupus patient uses a wheelchair
- minor adjustment in working hours if the lupus patient is required to rest due to fatigue.

"In the example of the schoolteacher cited above, the teacher with lupus was able to argue successfully that the school district could reasonably be asked to relieve her of her outdoor responsibilities. The lab technician was also able to argue that the lifting of heavy objects was not essential to her job responsibilities. The issue of her taking additional rest breaks is more difficult. If the worker is able to complete her daily tasks on time, without undue hardship to the employer, then she may successfully argue that the employer must make an accommodation for her rest breaks.

"State legislation in such states as New York and California also makes discrimination on the basis of disability illegal. The importance of such legislation is to ensure that those who have health problems, and can work, should not be denied the opportunity to do so."

17

The Lupus Foundation of America, Inc.: A Foundation with a Heart*

The Lupus Foundation of America, Inc. (LFA) was incorporated on November 11, 1977, and in only a few years it has become a major health organization with a membership of 25,000. Our national publication, *Lupus News*, reaches 50,000 readers.

Chapters of the Lupus Foundation of America have been formed in almost every state of the nation. Each chapter is composed of lupus patients and their families and is governed by a lay and medical advisory board. Together, the health-care professionals, the patients, their families, and lay leaders plan activities for the chapters. These activities increase awareness of lupus and help raise funds for medical research, educational programs, and patients' needs.

The LFA is a nonprofit patient-oriented organization, established in a society that is undergoing rapid medical and technological changes. The foundation's growth points to a new direction in medicine, derived from the experiences and special needs of persons afflicted with long-term disease.

As explained in previous chapters, lupus patients deal with a broad

* Ann Landers's description of the LFA in her popular column.

range of humane and ethical issues, including the impact of the disease on quality of life and on their interpersonal relationships. The foundation is particularly sensitive to these needs, and it helps the patient maintain a sense of worthiness.

Modern medicine has been revolutionized in the past few decades. New scientific knowledge has made possible open-heart surgery, kidney transplants, and even "test-tube" babies. But in the midst of the intensive search for still more scientific breakthroughs, many physicians have lost sight of the patients and seem to have less and less time to deal with humanistic considerations or to sort out the unique value of each human being.

Dr. Elizabeth Cole of Newton-Wellesley Hospital believes that high-technology medicine and high-technology practitioners often abandon empathy with patients in favor of a fascination with instruments. She stresses that while technology has been responsible for significant gains in health care, patients still need a relationship with their doctor that permits their fears and concerns to be appropriately managed. The psychological atmosphere that a physician creates, Dr. Cole says, can be as critical to a patient's recovery and satisfaction as the latest in diagnostic hardware.

The LFA is demonstrating some concern with such issues by stressing empathy with patients and concern for the social consequences of disease. Through public awareness and education, the foundation is encouraging preventive care for lupus patients rather than just crisis-oriented intervention. Physicians must be made aware of the need for education about the mortality of lupus. The issue of dying is very real to the patient, for the disease is often presented in the literature as rare and fatal. And while concerns about mortality are part of living with lupus and a major worry among lupus patients, for some of them the thought of dying becomes a preoccupation. Lupus patients should be helped to understand that, in most cases, death from lupus is not imminent, and patients and those close to them must learn to hope through education and understanding.

Directly relevant to the objectives of the Lupus Foundation of America are ongoing studies of the structure and function of the immune system and its disorders, under the purview of the National Institute of Allergy and Infectious Diseases (NIAID). Basic biomedical research and clinical investigations in the field of immunology are conducted in NIAID laboratories and clinics at the National

Institutes of Health in Bethesda, Maryland, and are supported by NIAID grants at university medical schools and centers throughout the country.

Taking advantage of its staff and institutional resources, NIAID has helped organize community-based projects designed to increase public and private awareness of the problems associated with lupus. Among the lectures and workshops undertaken in concert with NIAID-supported Allergic and Immunologic Disease Centers and local Lupus Foundation chapters and organized to enhance lupus awareness have been those of the following design:

- public programs for SLE patients and their families at the New York Hospital–Cornell Medical Center, cosponsored by Rockefeller and Cornell universities.
- workshops in SLE current concepts for physicians, at the Hospital of the Good Samaritan, cosponsored by the University of Southern California School of Medicine
- workshops on new horizons in research, diagnosis, and treatment of SLE at the Stanford (Calif.) University Medical Center
- community conferences on SLE for patients, families, concerned public, and health-care professionals—some bilingual (in English and Spanish)—at the University of Southern California–Los Angeles County Medical Center and the University of California, San Francisco Medical Center

Two particularly innovative programs were Chronicare '84, a model program and curriculum for community-based nurses on the care of patients with chronic disease formulated for nine weekly sessions (from February 1 to March 28, 1984, at the Newton-Wellesley School of Nursing and at Tufts University–New England Medical Center), and a workshop on immunologically relevant diseases at Boston's Children's Hospital.

Based on the success of and enthusiastic response to these programs, Dr. Sheldon Cohen, director of the NIAID Immunology, Allergic and Immunologic Disease Program, and his staff are planning to continue these endeavors as ongoing projects. Several LFA chapters have enthusiastically sought the opportunity to develop similar relationships with nearby university medical centers.* For more information, write: The Lupus Foundation, 11921A Olive Blvd., St. Louis, MO 63141.

Many lupus patients have joined the LFA because they feel isolated and stressed, and the lupus self-help groups offer settings where patients can share their concerns. Patients have reported a great sense of relief after being able to talk about their illness in the presence of people who can understand and respond with compassion. Patients whose affliction is mild often become a source of inspiration for patients who are not doing so well—and derive satisfaction from the realization that they are helping others.

Joan Marx, a psychotherapist from Brookline, Massachusetts, stresses that self-help and peer-support groups of similarly diagnosed patients can mean the difference between loneliness and friendship, between loss of self-esteem and establishing a new, improved sense of self for the lupus patient: "As a psychotherapist specializing in the treatment of chronically ill persons, I find my lupus patients often in need of peer support. While self-help groups cannot be a substitute for professional counseling, such groups, when properly structured, can be an invaluable source of emotional support and information.

"Meeting with friends who are waging the same battles, and meeting the same daily challenges, can reduce feelings of isolation and helplessness. Comparing symptoms and exchanging medical information can increase self-awareness, make more understandable a puzzling or seemingly uncontrollable condition, and broaden knowledge of available resources. For the newly diagnosed patient, talking with others who have lupus can make accepting and adjusting to a life with chronic illness less traumatic and frightening.

"The emotional and informational exchange that occurs among lupus peers in a self-help group transmits the single most valuable message to those in need of relief: 'You are not alone.' "

On behalf of that purpose, the LFA has established the following goals:

---

* A description of NIAID's community outreach program has appeared in *Lupus News*, Summer 1984.

1. to develop support for research programs designed to discover the cause(s) of and improve the methods of treating lupus

2. to promote understanding of the social and human costs imposed by lupus

3. to educate the patients and their families about lupus and offer them moral assistance and encouragement

4. to promote among physicians and other health professionals an exchange of knowledge with respect to lupus, and to cooperate with physicians and other health professionals in their efforts to improve the quality of life of the lupus patient

5. to represent lupus patients in forums both public and private

6. to encourage the creation of and cooperation among local chapters dedicated to serving lupus patients

The list beginning on page 209 gives addresses for chapters in the United States and other countries around the world.

ALABAMA

Birmingham Chapter
Lupus Foundation of America
924A 26th St., So.
Birmingham, AL 35205
205/252-3068

Montgomery Chapter
Lupus Foundation of America
P.O. Box 11507
Montgomery, AL 36111
205/288-3032

ARIZONA

Lupus Foundation of America
Greater Arizona Chapter, Inc.
5620 W. Thunderbird B-2
Glendale, AZ 85306
602/938-3302

ARKANSAS

Fort Smith Chapter
Lupus Foundation of America
P.O. Box 3863
Fort Smith, AR 72913
501/452-4571

CALIFORNIA

Bay Area Lupus Foundation,
  Inc.
265 Meridian Ave., Suite #5
San Jose, CA 95126
408/280-7616

Greater Los Angeles Chapter
Lupus Foundation of America
3741 Wasatch Avenue
Los Angeles, CA 90066
213/391-7774

Lupus Foundation of America
Greater San Gabriel Valley
  Chapter
P.O. Box 251
West Covina, CA 91793
818/332-3008

CONNECTICUT

Lupus Foundation of America
Connecticut Chapter, Inc.
P.O. Box 7-T
West Hartford, CT 06107
203/521-9151

COLORADO

Lupus Foundation of Colorado
P.O. Box 22621
Denver, CO 80222
303/758-0538

FLORIDA

Suncost Chapter
Lupus Foundation of America
2005 Healy Drive
Clearwater, FL 33575
813/733-5327

North Florida Lupus Foundation
P.O. Box 10486
Jacksonville, FL 32207
904/733-6472

Dade-Boward Lupus Foundation
  of Florida, Inc.
P.O. Box 4131
Miami, FL 33269-1131
305/653-1004

Florida Big Bend Chapter
Lupus Foundation of America
2118 Autumn Lane
Tallahassee, FL 32304
904/575-4497

Tampa Chapter
Lupus Foundation of America
305 South Hyde Park Ave.
Tampa, FL 33606
813/253-0620

Lupus Foundation of Palm
  Beach County, Inc.
P.O. Box 948
West Palm Beach, FL 33402
305/968-8827

Volusia Chapter
Lupus Foundation of America
P.O. Box 1858
Daytona Beach, FL 32015
904/734-0934

Lupus Foundation of Florida,
  Inc.
4121 N. Fort Christmas Road
Christmas, FL 32709
305/568-4303

Lupus Foundation of Pensacola
P.O. Box 17841
Pensacola, FL 32522
904/434-4551

GEORGIA

Lupus Foundation of America
  Greater Atlanta Chapter
2814 New Spring Rd., Rm.
  304A
Atlanta, GA 30339
404/432-9675

L.F.A. Augusta Chapter
2804 Sturnidae Court
Augusta, GA 30906
404/798-4894

L.F.A. Columbus Chapter
3911 Steam Mill Rd., Apt. J-11
Columbus, GA 31907
404/689-5795

ILLINOIS

L.E. Society of Illinois
P.O. Box 812
Chicago, IL 60642
312/779-3181

INDIANA

Indiana Lupus Foundation, Inc.
2701 E. Southport Road
Indianapolis, IN 46227
317/783-6033

Lupus Foundation of America
Northeast Indiana Chapter
% Mr. Jerry A. Young
P.O. Box 10581
Fort Wayne, IN 46853
219/432-9827

IOWA

Lupus Foundation of America
Iowa Chapter
P.O. Box 1723
Ames, IA 50010
515/232-3083

Eastern Iowa Chapter, LFA
1303 E. Davenport
Iowa City, IA 52240
319/351-1648

KANSAS

Lupus Foundation of Kansas
Wichita Chapter
P.O. Box 18742
Wichita, KS 67218
316/524-4973

Mr. Max Benjamin
Lupus Foundation of America
Kansas City Chapter
8831 Ensley Lane
Leawood, KS 66206
913/648-5984

KENTUCKY

Lupus Foundation of
  Kentuckiana, Inc.
2210 Goldsmith Ln., Suite 209
Louisville, KY 40218
502/459-6554

LOUISIANA

Louisiana Lupus Foundation
7732 Goodwood Blvd., Suite B
Baton Rouge, LA 70806
504/927-8052

Northeast Louisiana Chapter
Lupus Foundation of America
P.O. Box 7693
Monroe, LA 71201
318/325-5286

Lupus Foundation of America,
  Inc.
Cenla Chapter
P.O. Box 12565
Alexandria, LA 71315-2565
318/473-0125

Shreveport Chapter
Lupus Foundation of America
1961 Bayou Drive
Shreveport, LA 71105
318/861-2838

MAINE

Lupus Group of Maine
Eula Chrissiko
43 Settler Rd.
So. Portland, ME 04106
207/774-9219 or 774-2595

MARYLAND

The Maryland Lupus
  Foundation
12 West 25th Street
Baltimore, MD 21218
301/366-7272

MASSACHUSETTS

Lupus Foundation of America
Massachusetts Chapter
88 Tremont Street
Boston, MA 02108
617/523-8266

MICHIGAN

Michigan Lupus Foundation
19001 E. Eight Mile Road
East Detroit, MI 48021
313/775-8310

MINNESOTA

Minnesota Chapter
Lupus Foundation of America
640 11th Avenue South
Hopkins, MN 55343
612/933-4137

MISSISSIPPI

Lupus Foundation of America
Hattiesburg Chapter
P.O. Box 394
Petal, MS 39465
601/583-1489

LFA Central Mississippi Chapter
1215 North President St.
Jackson, MS 39202
601/352-4606

MISSOURI

Missouri Chapter
Lupus Foundation of America
8420 Delmar Blvd., Suite LL1
St. Louis, MO 63124
314/432-0008

MONTANA

Great Falls Lupus Chapter
% Ms. Ruby Peterson
R.R. 2833
Great Falls, MT 59401
406/454-1116

NEBRASKA

Lupus Foundation of America
Omaha Chapter
P.O. Box 14036
Omaha, NE 68124
402/333-9128

L.F.A. Western Nebraska
  Chapter
Beverly French
Box 12
Mullen, NE 69152
308/546-2518

NEVADA

Lupus Foundation of America
Northern Nevada Chapter
480 Galleti Way, Bldg. 14
Sparks, NV 89431
702/323-2444

LFA Las Vegas Chapter
2217 Santa Rosa Drive
Las Vegas, NV 89104
702/369-0474

NEW HAMPSHIRE

New Hampshire Lupus
  Foundation
% Thomas A. Mullin
P.O. Box 658
Durham, NH 03824
603/424-5668

NEW JERSEY

Lupus Foundation of America
South Jersey Chapter
P.O. Box 2101
Cherry Hill, NJ 08034
609/354-1234

Lupus Erythematosus
  Foundation of New Jersey
P.O. Box 320
Elmwood Park, NJ 07407
201/791-7868

NEW YORK

S.L.E. Foundation, Inc.
95 Madison Avenue, Suite 1402
New York, NY 10016
212/685-4118

Lupus Foundation of America
Genesee Valley Chapter
% Caroline Turner
18 Pecos Circle
West Henrietta, NY 14586
716/334-7209

Lupus Erythematosus Foundation
    Brooklyn Chapter, LFA
645 E. 85 St.
Brooklyn, NY 11236
212/241-6179

Lupus Foundation of America
Northeastern NY Chapter
2140 Broadway
Schenectady, NY 12306
518/393-3496

Lupus Foundation of America
Long Island/Queens Chapter
P.O. Box 236
Seaford, NY 11783
516/541-5088

Lupus Foundation of America
Central New York Chapter
423 W. Onondaga Street
Syracuse, NY 13202
315/471-7788

Lupus Foundation of America
NY Southern Tier Chapter
Suite 337 N Press Bldg.
19 Chenango St.
Binghamton, NY 13901
607/772-6522

Lupus Foundation of America
Rockland & Orange Chapter
Martha MacRobbie
14 Kingston Drive
Spring Valley, NY 10977
914/254-0372

Lupus Foundation of America
Western New York Chapter
250 Athens Blvd.
Tonawanda, NY 14223
716/835-7161

Lupus Foundation of America
Marguerite Curri Chapter
P.O. Box 853
Utica, NY 13503
315/732-4291

Westchester Lupus Foundation
P.O. Box 133
Valhalla, NY 10595
914/948-1032

NORTH CAROLINA

Blueridge Chapter
Lupus Foundation of America
1763 Highland Ave., NE
Hickory, NC 28601
704/328-4798

Lupus Foundation of America
Raleigh Chapter
% John Essen
601 N. Main St.
Graham, NC 27253
919/227-1604

Lupus Foundation of America
Winston Triad Chapter
% Ms. Ruth Banbury
2841 Foxwood Lane
Winston-Salem, NC 27103
919/768-1493

Lupus Foundation of America
Charlotte Chapter
2401 Thornridge Road
Charlotte, NC 28226
704/399-3761

OHIO

Lupus Foundation of America
Akron Area Chapter
American Red Cross Bldg.
501 W. Market Street
Akron, OH 44303
216/535-3761

Lupus Foundation of America
Greater Cleveland Chapter
P.O. Box 22319
Cleveland, OH 44122-0319
216/531-6563

Lupus Foundation of America
Columbus, OH, March Zitron
  Chapter
5180 East Main Street
Columbus, OH 43213
614/267-0811

Dayton Lupus Club
Mrs. Rose Bower, Pres.
5181 Pundt Rd.
Lewisburg, OH 45338
513/962-2887

Stark County Lupus Association
Rainbow Chapter
P.O. Box 1038
Massillon, OH 44648
216/833-4811

Youngstown Area Chapter
Lupus Foundation of America
4196 Adeer Drive
Canfield, OH 44406
216/743-5877

OKLAHOMA

Oklahoma Lupus Ass'n., Inc.
6521 N.W. 30th Terrace
Bethany, OK 73008
405/787-8223

Tulsa Chapter of the Oklahoma
  Lupus Association
% Ms. Cheryl Collins
  Thornburg
6421 S. 109th East Ave.
Tulsa, OK 74133
918/835-5483

PENNSYLVANIA

Lupus Foundation of
  Philadelphia, Inc.
5415 Claridge Street
Philadelphia, PA 19124
215/743-7171

Lupus Foundation of America
Ches-Mont Chapter
RD #1, Box 254
Pottstown, PA 19464
215/367-2264

Lupus Foundation of Delaware
  Valley, Inc.
Mrs. Robert Zeit
541 Jamestown Ave.
Philadelphia, PA 19128
215/642-8430 or 483-5445

Pennsylvania Lupus Foundation,
  Inc.
P.O. Box 264
Wayne, PA 19087
215/477-7020

Lupus Alert, Inc.
P.O. Box 8
Folsom, PA 19033
215/532-6771

Lupus Foundation of America
Western PA Chapter
3380 Blvd. of the Allies
Pittsburgh, PA 15213
412/647-3676

RHODE ISLAND

Lupus Foundation of America
Rhode Island Chapter
8 Fallon Avenue
Providence, RI 02908
401/421-7227

SOUTH CAROLINA

South Carolina Chapter
Lupus Foundation of America
P.O. Box 7511
Columbia, SC 29202
803/791-8471

TENNESSEE

Mountain Empire Chapter
Lupus Foundation of America
3132 Memorial Blvd.
Kingsport, TN 37664
615/246-5178

East Tennessee Chapter
5612 Kingston Pike, Suite 5
Knoxville, TN 37919
615/584-5215

Lupus Foundation of America
Memphis Area Chapter
5117 Scrivener
Memphis, TN 38134
901/377-2555 or 388-2090

TEXAS

Lupus Foundation of America
Dallas Chapter
% Ruth Fantus
P.O. Box 835914
Richardson, TX 75083
214/289-2344

El Paso Lupus Association
Northgate Center, Suite F
9348 Dyer
El Paso, TX 79924
915/755-8374

Lupus Foundation of America,
   Houston Chapter
Ms. Susan Berger
% Ernst & Whinney
333 Clay Street, Suite 3100
Houston, TX 77002
713/682-0497

San Antonio Area Lupus Fdn.
P.O. Box 17512
San Antonio, TX 78217
512/681-6057 or 654-9236

UTAH

Lupus Foundation of America
Northern Utah Chapter
P.O. Box 1677
Ogden, UT 84402
801/621-3748

VIRGINIA

Lupus Foundation of America
Central Virginia Chapter
P.O. Box 14507
Richmond, VA 23221-0507
804/262-9622

Lupus Foundation of America
Eastern Virginia Chapter
7404 Ocean Front
Virginia Beach, VA 23451
804/422-2862

Greater Washington Chapter
Lupus Foundation of America
7297-D Lee Highway
Falls Church, VA 22042
703/533-9852

WEST VIRGINIA

Lupus Foundation of America
Kanawha Valley Chapter of West
  Virginia
P.O. Box 8274
S. Charleston, WV 25303

The Lupus Foundation of West
  Virginia, Inc.
Mary Louise Menendez

4 Fleming St.
Shinnston, WV 26431
304/592-0015

WISCONSIN

L.E. Society of Wisconsin, Inc.
P.O. Box 16621
Milwaukee, WI 53216
414/781-1111

CANADA

Lupus Foundation of Ontario
% Mrs. Karen Glen
289 Ridge Road N
P.O. Box 687
Ridgeway, Ontario
Canada LOS 1NO
Phone: 416/894-4611

The Lupus Society of Hamilton
236 King Street W
Hamilton, Ontario
Canada L8P 1A9
Phone: 416/527-2252

Ontario Lupus Association
920 Yonge Street, Ste. 420
Toronto, Ontario
Canada M4W 3J7
Phone: 416/967-1414

References
and Selected Bibliography

Introduction: An Overview of Lupus

GLASS, DAVID and SCHUR, PETER H.: Autoimmunity and Systemic Lupus Erythematosus, In: *Autoimmunity Genetic, Immunologic, Virologic, and Clinical Aspects*, ed., Norman Talal, Academic Press, Inc., 1977, pp. 532–568.

GLASS, D., RAUM, D., GIBSON, D., STILLMAN, J.S. and SCHUR, P. H.: Inherited deficiency of the second component of complement. Rheumatic disease associations. *J. Clin. Invest.*, 58:853–861, 1976.

KOFLER, D., SCHUR, P. H. and KUNKEL, H. G.: Immunological studies concerning the nephritis of systemic lupus erythematosus. *J. Exp. Med.* 126:607–623, 1967.

PINCUS, P., SCHUR, P. H., ROSE, J. A., DECKER, J. L. and TALAL, N.: Measurement of serum DNA-binding activity in systemic lupus erythematosus. *New Eng. J. Med.* 281:701–707, 1969.

RAUM, D., GLASS, D., CARPENTER, C. B., ALPER, C. A. and SCHUR, P. H.: The chromosomal order of genes controlling the major histocompatibility complex, properdin factor B, and deficiency of the second component of complement. *J. Clin. Invest.* 58:1240–1248, 1976.

SCHUR, PETER H.: Lupus Erythematosus, In *Advances in Nephrology*, ed. Hamburger, J., Crosiner, J., and Maxwell, M. H., Yearbook Medical Publishers, Inc., 1976, pp. 63–77.

SCHUR, PETER H.: Pathophysiology of Rheumatic Diseases. *Arthritis and Rheumatism* 20:500–508, 1977.

SCHUR, P. H. and SANDSON. J.: Immunological factors and clinical activity in lupus erythematosus. *New Eng. J. Med.* 278:533–538, 1968.

SCHUR, P. H., STELLAR, B. D., STEINBERG, A. D. and TALAL, N.: Incidence of antibodies to double-stranded DNA in systemic lupus erythematosus and related diseases. *Arth. and Rheum.* 14:342–347, 1971.

SCHUR, P. H.: Systemic lupus erythematosus. In *Textbook of Medicine*, ed. Beeson and McDermott, W. B. Saunders Co., 1975, pp. 131–136.

SCHUR, P. H.: Complement in lupus. In *Clinics in Rheumatic Diseases, Systemic Lupus Erythematosus*, ed. N. F. Rothfield, vol. 1, W. B. Saunders Co., Ltd., London, p. 519–543, 1975.

SCHUR, P. (ed.) *The Clinical Management of Systemic Lupus Erythematosus*. Orlando, Florida. Grune and Stratton, 1983.

TAN, E. M., SCHUR, P. H., CARR, R. I. and KUNKEL, H. G.: DNA and antibodies to DNA in the serum of patients with systemic lupus erythematosus. *J. Clin. Invest.* 45:1732–1740, 1966.

Milestones in the History of Systemic Lupus Erythematosus

BAEHR, G., KLEMPERER, P., SCHIFRIN, A.: A diffuse disease of the peripheral circulation (usually associated with lupus erythematosus and endocarditis). *Trans Assoc Amer Phys* 50:139–155, 1935.

BAEHR, G., SOFFER, L. J.: Treatment of disseminated lupus erythematosus with cortisone and adrenocorticoatropin.. *Bull New York Acad Med* 26:229–234, 1950.

BAEHR, G., SOFFER, L., BOAR, N. F., LEVITT, M. F., GABRILOVE, J. L.: The influence of cortisome and adrenocorticotropin in disseminated lupus erythematosus. *Trans Assoc Amer Phys* 63:89–98, 1950.

HARGRAVES, M. M., RICHMOND, H., MORTON, R.: Presentation of two bone marrow elements: the "tart" cell and the "L.E." cell. *Proc Staff Meet Mayo Clin* 23:25–28, 1948.

KLEMPERER, P.: The concept of collagen diseases. *Am J Path* 26:505–519, 1950.

KLEMPERER, P., POLLACK, A. D., BAEHR, G.: Diffuse collagen disease. Acute disseminated lupus erythematosus and diffuse scleroderma. *JAMA* 119:331–332, 1942.

KLEMPERER, P., POLLACK, A. D., BAEHR, G.: Pathology of disseminated lupus erythematosus. *Arch Path* 32:569–631, 1941.

LIBMAN, E., SACKS, B.: A hitherto undescribed form of vascular and mural endocarditis. *Arch Intern Med* 33:701–737, 1924.

RODNAN, G. P.: Growth and development of rheumatology in the United States—a bicentennial report. Presidential address to the American Rheumatism Association. *Arthritis Rheum* 20:1149–1168, 1977.

1: Lupus and Epidemiology

BLOCK, S. R., WINFIELD, J. B., LOCKSHIN, M. D., D'ANGELO, W. A., CHRISTIAN, C. L.: Studies of twins with SLE—a review of literature and presentation of 12 additional sets, *Am J Med* 1975; 59:533–552.

FRIEDMAN, G. D.: *Primer of Epidemiology*. New York, McGraw-Hill, 1974.

HOOVER, R., FRAUMENI, J. F., JR.: *Risk of cancer in renal transplant recipients*. Lancet 1973; 2:55–57.

KASLOW, R. A., MASI, A. T.: Age, sex, and race effects on mortality from systemic lupus erythematosus in the United States. *Arth Rheum* 1978; 21:473–479.

REINERTSEN, J. R., KASLOW, R. A., KLIPPEL, J. H., et al: An epidemiologic study of households exposed to canine systemic lupus erythematosus. *Arth Rheum* 1980; 24:564–568.

SIEGEL, M., LEE, S. L.: The epidemiology of systemic lupus erythematosus. *Sem Arth Rheum* 1973; 3:1–54.

2: Lupus and Genetics

BENACERRAF, B., and UNANUE, E. R. *Textbook of Immunology*. Williams and Wilkins, Baltimore, 1979, 298 pp.

HARRIS, HARRY. *Principles of Human Biochemical Genetics*. Second edition. North-Holland, Amsterdam, 1975.

KAN, Y. W., and DOZY, A. M. Polymorphism of DNA sequence adjacent to human B-globin structural gene: relationship to sickle mutation. *Proc. Natl. Acad. Sci. U.S.A. 75*: 5631–5635.

REINERTSEN, J. L., KLIPPEL, J. H. JOHNSON, A. H., STEINBERG, A. D., DECKER, J. L., and MANN, D. L., B-Lymphocyte Antigens Associated with Systemic Lupus Erythematosus, *New England Journal of Medicine* 299:575, 1978.

3: Research in Systemic Lupus Erythematosus

Unraveling some of the Mysteries of Lupus
Anonymous Binding of synthetic double stranded DNA by serum from patients with systemic lupus erythematosus: correlation with renal histology. Steinman, C. R., Grishman, E., Spiera, H. and Deesomchok, U. *Am. J. Med.* 62:319–323, 1977.

DAVIS, G. S. JR., and DAVIS, J. S., IV. Detection of circulating DNA by counterimmunoelectrophoresis (CIE). *Arthritis & Rheum.* 16:52–58, 1973.

Detection of anti DNA antibody using synthetic antigens. Steinman,

C. R. Deesomchok, V. and Spiera, H. J. Clin. Invest. 57:1330–1341, 1976.

Free DNA in serum and plasma from normal adults. C. R., J. Clin. Invest. 56:512–515, 1975.

GRISHMAN, E., PROUSH., J. G., LEE, S. L., CHURG, J., Renal biopsies in lupus nephritis. Correlation of electronmicroscopic findings with clinical course. Nephron 10:25, 1973.

LEVINE, L. and STOLLAR, B. D. Nucleic acid immune systems. Prog. Allergy 12:161–191, 1968.

STEINMAN, C. R. Circulating DNA in systemic lupus erythematosus. Association with central nervous system involvement and systemic vasculitis. Am. J. Med. 67:429–435, 1979.

TAN, E. M., SCHUR, P. H., CARR, R. I. and KUNKEL, H. G. Deoxyribonucleic acid (DNA) and antibodies to DNA in the serum of patients with systemic lupus erythematosus. Jclin Invest. 45:1732–1740, 1966.

Suppressor T Cells

GLADMAN, D., KEYSTONE, E., UROURTZ, M., CANE, D., and POPLONSKI, L. Impaired Antigen-Specific Suppressor Cell Activity in Patients with Systemic Lupus Erythematosus, Clin. Exp. Immunol. 40:77, 1980.

HERZENBERG, L. A., BLACK, S. J., and HERZENBERG, L. A. Regulatory Circuits and Antibody Response, Europ. J. of Immunol. 10:1, 1980.

WALDMANN, T. A., and BRODER, S. Suppressor cells in the Regulation of the Immune Response in Progress in Clinical Immunology, Schwarz, R. S. (editor) 3:155, 1977.

Transmissible Factors in SLE?

CARR, R. J., HOFFMAN, A. E., and HARBECK, R. J., Comparison of DNA Binding in the Normal Population, General Hospital Laboratory Personnel and Personnel From Laboratories Studying SLE, J. Rheumatol. 2:178, 1975.

DEHORATIUS, R. J., and MESNER, R. P., Lymphocytotoxic Antibodies in Family Members of Patients with Systemic Lupus Erythematosus, J. Clin. Invest. 55:1254, 1975.

LOWENSTEIN, M. B., and ROTHFIELD, N. D., Family Study of Systemic Lupus Erythematosus, Arthritis and Rheumatism 20:1293, 1977.

Food-Induced Immune Tolerance

HANSON, D. G., VAZ, N. M., MAIA, L. C. S., HORNBROOK, M. N., LYNCH, J. M., and ROY, C. A. Inhibition of Specific Immune Responses by Feeding Protein Antigens, Int. Arch. Allergy and Applied Immunology 55:526, 1977.

RICHMAN, L. K., CHILLER, J. M., BROWN, W. R., HANSON, D. G., and VAZ, N. M. Enterically induced Immunologic Tolerance, *J. Immunology*, 121:2429, 1978.

SWARBRICK, E. T., STOKES, C. R., and SOOTHILL, J. F. Absorption of Antigens After Oral Immunization and the Simultaneous Induction of Specific Systemic Tolerance, *Gut* 20:121, 1979.

WALKER, W. A. and ISSELBACHER, K. J., Uptake and Transport of Macromolecules by the Intestine. Possible role in Clinical disorders, *Gastroenterology* 67:531, 1975.

Ingested Antigens May Play a Role
in The Pathogenesis of SLE

DECKER, J. L., STEINBERG, A. D., REINERTSEN, J. L., PLOTZ, P. H., BALOW, J. E., and KLIPPEL, J. H. Systemic Lupus Erythematosus: *Evolving Concepts, Annals of Internal Medicine*, 91:587, 1979.

DUBOIS, E. L. Lupus Erythematosus, 2nd Ed. (revised, University of Southern California Press), 1976.

ZURIER, R. B., Systemic Lupus Erythematosus, Hospital Practice, August, 1979.

IgA Deficiency, Increased Autoimmunity
and Increased Levels of Antibodies to Food Antigens

AMMANN, A. J., and HONG, R. Selective IgA Deficiency: Presentation of 30 Cases and a Review of the Literature, *Medicine* 50:223, 1971.

CARR, RONALD I., WOLD, R. T., and FARR, R. S. Antibodies to Bovine Gammaglobulin (BGG) and the Occurrence of a BGG-like Substance in Systemic Lupus Erythematosus (SLE) sera, *J. Allergy and Clin. Immunol.* 50:18, 1972.

CUNNINGHAM, RUNDLES, C., BRANDEIS, W. E., GOOD, R. A., and DAY, N. K. Bourne Antigens and the Formation of Circulating Immune Complexes in Selective Immunoglobulin A Deficiency.

PETERSON, R. D., and GOOD, R. A. Antibodies to Cow's Milk Proteins: Their presence and significance. *Pediatrics* 31:209, 1963.

BARRETT, D. J., BERTANI, L., WARA, DIANE W., AMMANN, A. J. Milk precipitins in selective IgA deficiency, *Annals of Allergy*, 42:73, 1979.

Dogs and Lupus

LEWIS, R. M., SCHWARTZ, R. S., HENRY, W. B. Canine systemic lupus erythematosus, *Blood*, 25:143 (1965).

LEWIS, ROBERT M., TANNENBERG, WALTER, EMILLOWITZ, CHRISTINA, SCHWARTZ, ROBERT S. et al, C-type viruses in SLE, *Nature*, 1974, pp. 152, 78 No. 547.2, pp. 78–99, No. 1, 1977.

LEWIS, R. M., SCHWARTZ, J. A., HARRIS, G. S., HIRSCH, M. S., BLACK, P. H., SCHWARTZ, R. S. Canine Systemic Lupus Erythematosus: Transmission of Serologic Abnormalities by Cellfree Filtrates, *Journal of Clinical Investigation*, 52:1893 (1973).

LEWIS, R. M., SCHWARTZ, R. S. Canine Systemic Lupus Erythematosus: Genetic Analysis of an established breeding colony, *Journal of Experimental Medicine*, 134:417 (1971).

MARK, D. A., ALONSO, D. R., QUIMBY, F. W., THALER, H. T., KIM, Y. T., FERNANDES, G., GOOD, R. A. and WEKSLER, M. E. Effects of Nutrition on Disease and Life Span: I. Effects on Immune responses, cardiovascular pathology and life span in MRL mice. *Amer. J. Pathol.*, 1984 (in press).

QUIMBY, F., GEBERT R., DATTA, S., ANDRE-SCHWARTZ, J., GANNENBERG, W., LEWIS, R. M., WEINSTEIN, I. and SCHWARTZ, R. S.: Isolation and characterization of a retrovirus associated with canine and human SLE. *Clin. Immunol. Immunopath.* 9:194–210, 1978.

QUIMBY, F. W., and SCHWARTZ, R. S.: Etiopathogenesis of Systemic lupus erythematosus. In: Pathobiology Annual 1978, 8:35–59. H. L. Ioachin (Editor) Raven Press, New York.

QUIMBY, F. W., JENSEN, C., NEWROCKI, D. and SCOLLIN, P.: Selected Autoimmune Diseases in the Dog. In: V*et. Clinics of North America* 8:32–38, 1978.

QUIMBY, F. W., SCHWARTZ, R. S., POSKITT, T. and LEWIS, R. M. 1979. A disorder of dogs resembling Sjogren's Syndrome. *Clin. Immunol. Immunopath.* 12:471.

QUIMBY, F. W., DRUSHWEIN, M., SMITH, C. and LEWIS, R. M. 1980. The efficacy of Immunoserodiagnostic procedures in the recognition of canine immunologic diseases. *Am. J. Vet. Res.* 41:1662–1666, 1980.

QUIMBY, F. W., and PICCOLIE, A.: A syndrome resembling thyrogastric disease in a dog. Presented at the 29th annual session, American Assoc. for Lab. Animal S ience, New York, 1978.

QUIMBY, F. W. and ZiNK, N.: Autoimmunity, multiple primary neoplasia and liver disease in a family of dogs. Presented at the 29th annual session of Am. Assoc. Lab. Animal Sci., 1978.

SCHWARTZ, R. S., QUIMBY, P., ANDRE-SCHWARTZ, J.: Canine systemic lupus erythematosus. Phenotypic expression of autoimmunity in a closed colony. In Genetic Control of Autoimmune Disease. (N.R. Rose et al, editors), Elsevier-North Holland, Inc., New York, 1979, in press.

4: Why Lupus is More Common in Women than in Men

Arthritis and Rheumatism, Official Journal of the American Rheumatism Association Section of the Arthritis Foundation.

Differentiation of the Immune Response—"High Sensitivity to Androgen as a Contributing Factor in Sex Differences in the Immune Response," D. A. Cohn, p. 1218. "Effect of Estrogen on Natural Killer Cells," William E. Seaman and Thomas D. Gindhart, p. 1234. "The Role of the Endocrine Thymus in Female Reproduction," Sandra D. Michael, p. 1241. "Glucocorticoids and Immune Responses," Gerald R. Crabtree. Steven Gillis, Kendall A. Smith, and Allan Nunch, p. 1246.

H-Y Antigens—"Primary Sex Determination: H-Y Antigen and the Development of the Mammalian Testis," Stephen S. Wachtel, p. 1200. "Identification of Human H-Y antigen and its Testis-Organizing Function," Hikaru Iwata, Yukifumi Nagai, Dwight D. Stapleton, Richard C. Smith, and Susumu Ohno, p. 1211.

Immune Response to Viruses—"Sex Differences in Response to Hepatitis B Virus," Introduction, p. 1258, W. Thomas London; I. History, p. 1261, II. Parental Responses to HBV Infection and the Secondary Sex Ratio of the Offspring, Baruch S. Blumberg, p. 1264; III. Responses to HBV and Sex of Donor and Recipient in Kidney and Bone Marrow Transplantation, W. Thomas London, p. 1267.

Proceedings of the Kroc Foundation Conference on Sex Factors, Steroid Hormones, and the Host Response, Santa Ynez Valley, California, February 12–16, 1979. Editor, Norman Talal, M.D., Vol. 22, No. 11, November, 1979.

Sex Factors and Autoimmunity—"Sex Hormone Modulation of Autoimmunity in NZB/NZW Mice," Jirayr Roubinian, Norman Talal, Pentti K. Siiteri and Jacqueline A. Sadakian, p. 1162. "Approach to the Study of the Role of Sex Hormones in Autoimmunity," Alfred D. Steinberg, Kathleen A. Melez, Elizabeth S. Raveche, J. Patton Reeves, William A. Boegel, Patricia A. Smathers, Joel D. Taurog, Lisa Weinlein, and Madeleine Duvic, p. 1170. "Studies of the Effects of Sex Hormones on Autosomal and X-Linked Genetic Control of Induced and Spontaneous Antibody Production," E. S. Raveche, J. H. Tijo, W. Boegel, and A. D. Steinberg, p. 1177. "A Y Chromosome Associated Factor in Strain BXSB Producing Accelerated Autoimmunity and Lymphoproliferation," Edwin D. Murphy and John B. Roths, p. 1188. "Alterations of Estrogen Metabolism in Systemic Lupus Erythematosus," Robert G. Lahita, H. Leon Bradlow, Henry G. Kunkel, and Jack Fishman, p. 1195.

Sex Hormones, Pregnancy, and the Immune Response—"The Mechanism of Phenotypic Sex Differentiation," Jean D. Wilson, James E. Griffin, and Fredrick W. George, p. 1275. "Sex Hormone Production and Action," Pentti K. Siiteri, p. 1284. "Effect of Sex Hormones on the Complement-Related Clinical Disorder of Hereditary Angioedema," Michael M. Frank, p. 1295. "Immunologic Regulation in Pregnancy," Daniel P. Stites, Charles S. Pavia, Louis E. Clemens, Robert W. Kuhn, and

Pentti K. Siiteri, p. 1300. "Placenta-Bound Immunoglobulins," Abdo Jurjus, David A. Wheeler, Robert C. Gallo, and Isaac P. Witz, p. 1308.

6: Lupus and Medications

BALDWIN, D. S. et al: The clinical course of the proliferative and membranous forms of lupus nephritis, *Ann. Intern. Med.* 73:929, 1970.

BARNETT, E. V., DORNFELD, L., LEE, D. LIEBLING, M. (1978) Long-term survival of lupus nephritis patients treated with azathioprine and prednisone. *Journal of Rheumatology*, 5(3), 275.

CADE, R., SPOONER, G., SCHLEIN, E., et al (1973) Comparison of azathioprine, prednisone and heparin alone or combined in treating lupus nephritis. *Nephron*, 10,37.

CATHCART, E. S., IDELSON, B. A., SCHEINBERG, A., COUSER, W. B. (1976) Beneficial effects of methylprednisolone 'pulse' therapy in diffuse proliferative lupus nephritis. *Lancet*, i, 163–165.

DECKER, J. L. et al: Systemic lupus crythematosus: contrasts and comparisons, *Ann. Intern. Med.* 82:391, 1975.

DECKER, J. L. et al: Cyclophosphamide or azathioprine in lupus glomerulonephritis, *Ann. Intern. Med.* 83:606, 1975.

DONADIO, J. V., HOLLEY, K. E., WAGANER, R. D. et al. (1974) Further observation on the treatment of lupus nephritis with prednisone and combined prednisone and azathioprine. *Arthritis and Rheumatism*, 17, 573.

DONADIO, J. V. (1977) Treatment of Lupus nephritis. *Nephron*, 19, 186–189.

DONADIO, J. V., JR., HOLLEY, K. E., FERGUSON, R. H., ILSTRUP. D. M. (1978) Treatment of diffuse proliferative lupus nephritis with prednisone and combined prednisone and cyclophosphamide. *New England Journal of Medicine*, 299, 115, 1978.

DUBOIS, E. L. (1974) Lupus Erythematosus. U.S.C. Press.

DUBOIS, E. L. (1978) Antimalarials in the management of discoid and systemic lupus erythematosus. *Seminars in Arthritis and Rheumatism*, 8, 33–51.

EPSTEIN, R. H. et al: Case 2-1976 (Case Records of the Massachusetts General Hospital), *N. Eng. J. Med.* 294:100, 1976.

PHILLIPS, P. E.: The virus hypothesis in systemic lupus erythematosus, *Ann. Intern. Med.* 83:709, 1975.

GINZLER, E., DIAMOND, H., GUTTACAURIA, M., KAPLAN. D. (1976) Prednisone and azathioprine compared to prednisone treatment of diffuse lupus nephritis. *Arthritis and Rheumatism*, 19, 693–699.

HAHN, B. H., KANTOR, O. S., OSTERLAND, C. K.: Azathioprine plus prednisone compared with prednisone alone in the treatment of systemic lupus erythematosus, *Ann. Intern. Med.* 83:597, 1975.

HUGHES, G. R. V. (1979) The treatment of systemic lupus erythematosus: The case for conservative management. *Chapter in Clinics in Rheumatic Diseases on Anti-Rheumatic Drugs* 5, 2.

HUSKISSON, E. C. Editor (1979) Anti-rheumatic Drugs. *Clinics in Rheumatic Diseases* 5, 2.

KAPLAN, S. R., CALABRESI, P. (1973) Cytotoxic drugs in non-neoplastic diseases. *Part I & II New England Journal of Medicine*, 289, 952–955 & 1234–1236.

KIMBERLY, R. P., PLOTZ, P. H. (1977) Aspirin-induced depression of renal function. *New England Journal of Medicine*, 296, 418.

PAULUS, H. E. and FURST, D. E. (1979) Chapter on Aspirin and Nonsteroidal Anti-inflammatory drugs in Arthritis and Allied Conditions. Ed. D. J. McCarty, Lea and Febiger.

POLLAK, V. E. (1976) Treatment of lupus nephritis. *Advances in Nephrology*, 6, 137–161.

ROPES, MARIAN W., M.D., *Systemic Lupus Erythematosus.* Boston: Harvard University Press, 1976.

RUDNICK, R. D., GRESHAM, G. E., ROTHFIELD, N. F. (1975) The efficacy of antimalarials in systemic lupus erythematosus. *Journal of Rheumatology*, 2:323–330, 1975.

SCHEINBERG, M. A., CATHCART, E. S., GOLDSTEIN, A. L.: Thymosin-induced reduction of "null cells" in peripheral blood lymphocytes of patients with systemic lupus erythematosus, *Lancet* 1:424, 1975.

SEAMAN, W. E. ISHAK, K. G., PLOTZ, P. E. (1974) Aspirin-induced hepatotoxicity in patients with SLE, *Annals of Internal Medicine*, 80, 1–8.

SEAMAN, W. E., POLOTZ, P. H. (1976) Effect of aspirin on liver tests in patients with RA or SLE and in normal volunteers. *Arthritis and Rheumatism*, 19, 155–160.

SONNENBLICK, M., ABRAHAM, A. S. (1978) Ibuprofen sensitivity in SLE. *British Medical Journal*, i, 619–620.

URMAN, J. D., ROTHFIELD, N. F. (1977) Corticosteroid treatment in systemic lupus erythematosus: survival studies. *Journal of the American Medical Association*, 238, 2272.

WILSON, W., HUGHES, G. R. V. (1976) Immunosuppressives in the rheumatic diseases. Ropics in Rheumatology, ed. Hughes, G. R. V., London. Heineman.

ZURIER, R. B., S. HOFFSTEIN, G. WEISSMANN, "Suppression of Acute and Chronic Inflammation in Adrenalectomized rate by Pharmacologic amounts of Prostaglandins," *Arthritis and Rheumatism*, 16:606, 1973.

ZURIER, R. B., "Prostaglandins, Inflammation and Asthma," *Arch. Intern. Med.*, 133:101–110, 1974.

7: Lupus and Photosensitivity

BAER, R. L., HARBER, L. C.: Photobiology of lupus erythematosus. *Arch Dermatol* 92:124–128, 1965.

CRIPPS, D. J., RANKIN, J.: Action spectra of lupus erythematosus and experimental immunofluorescence. *Arch Dermatol* 107:563–567, 1973.

DILAIMY, M.: Lichen planus subtropicus. *Arch Dermatol* 112:1251–1253, 1976.

EPSTEIN, J. H., et al: Light sensitivity and lupus erythematosus. *Arch Dermatol* 91:483–485, 1965.

FREEMAN R. G., et al: Cutaneous lesions of lupus erythematosus induced by monochromatic light. *Arch Dermatol* 100: 677–682, 1969.

MANDULA, B. B., PATHAK, M. A.: Metabolic reactions in vitro of psoralens with liver and epidermis. *Biochemical Pharmacology.* Vol 28:127–132, 1979.

MANDULA, B. B., PATHAK, M. A.: Photochemotherapy, identification of a metabolite of 4, 5', 8-trimethyl psoralen. *Science,* Vol 193:1131–1134, 1976.

MATHEWS-ROTH, M. M., PATHAK, M. A., FITZPATRICK, T. B., HARBOR, L. C., KASS, E. H.: Beta carotene as a photoprotective agent in erythropoietic protoporphyria. *New England Journal Med.* 282:1231–1234, 1970.

NATALI, P. G., and TAN, E. M.: Experimental skin lesions in mice resembling systemic lupus erythematosus, *Arthritis Rheum.* 16:579, 1973.

NATALI, P. G., et al.: Effect of complement and polymorphonuclear leukocyte depletion on experimental skin lesions resembling systemic lupus erythematosus, *Arthritis Rheum.* 18:581, 1975.

O'QUINN, S. E., et al: Problems of disability in patients with chronic skin diseases, *Arch Dermatol.* Vol 105:35, 1972.

PATHAK, M. A. FITZPATRICK, T. B., PARRISH, J. A.: Photosensitivity and other reactions to light. In Harrison's *Principles of Internal Medicine,* 9th Ed., K. J. Isselbacher, et al eds., McGraw Hill Book Co. N.Y., 1979, Chapter 55, pp. 255–262.

PATHAK, M. A., JIMBO, K., FITZPATRICK, T. B.: Photobiology of the pigment cell. In *Phenotypic Expression in Pigment Cells.* Ed M. Seiji, Univ. of Tokyo Press, Tokyo, Japan, 1981, pp. 655–670.

PATHAK, M. A., EPSTEIN, J. H.: Normal and abnormal reactions of man to light. In *Dermatology in General Medicine:* 1st Ed. (Fitzpatrick, T. B., et al). McGraw Hill Book Co. New York. Chapter 17, pp. 977–1036, 1971.

PATHAK, M. A., FITZPATRICK, T. B.: Photosensitivity Caused by Drugs. *Rational Drug Therapy.* 6:1–6, 1972.

PATHAK, M. A., KRAMER, D. M., FITZPATRICK, T. B.: Photobiology & photochemistry of furocoumarins (psoralen). *Sunlight & Man: Normal and Abnormal Photobiologic Responses.* Pathak, M. A., et al eds., Univ. of Tokyo Press, Tokyo, Japan, 1974, pp. 335–369.

PATHAK, M. A., KRAMER, D. M., FITZPATRICK, T. B.: The role of natural photoprotection agents in human skin. *Ibid.*, pp. 725–751.

PATHAK, M. A., JIMBO, K., SZABO, G., FITZPATRICK, T. B.: Sunlight and melanopigmentation. In Photochemical and Photobiological Reviews. K. C. Smith, ed., Plenum Press. N.Y., 1976, pp. 211–239.

PATHAK, M. A., STRATTON, K.: A study of the free radicals in human skin before and after exposure to light. *Arch. Bio. Chem. Bio. Phys.* 123:468–476, 1968.

PATHAK, M. A., KRAMER, D. M.: Photosynthesization of the skin in vivo by furocoumarins (psoralens). *Bio. Chim. Bio. Phys. Acta* 195:197–206, 1969.

PATHAK, M. A., FITZPATRICK, T. B., FRAENK, E.: Evaluation of topical agents that prevent sunburn. Superiority of para-amino benzoic acid and its ester in ethyl alcohol. *New England Journal Med.* 280:1459, 1969.

SCOTT, B. S., PATHAK, M. A., MOHN, G. R.: Molecular and genetic basis of furocoumarin reactions. *Mutation Research* 39:29–74, 1976.

TAN, E. M.: Immunopathology and pathogenesis of cutaneous involvement in systemic lupus erythematosus, *J. Invest. Dermatol.* 67:360, 1976.

TUFFANELLI, D. L.: Connective tissue diseases. In *The YearBook of Dermatology*, ed. Malkinson, F. D. et al., YearBook Medical Publishers, Inc., Chicago, 1978, pp. 9–36.

8: The Patient, the Physician, and the Psychiatrist

BALINT, MICHAEL, M.D., *The Doctor, the Patient, and His Illness.* New York: International Press, 1972.

NICOBION: *Literature uber die Therapeutische Anwendung der Nikot insareamidis.* Darmstadt, Germany: The Mirch Company, 1941, pp. 14–19.

POPOFF, L., POPCHRISTOFF, M., and BATCHVAROFF, B., *Bull. Soc. Franc. Dermat. Syph.* 46:1038–1041, 1939.

POPOFF, L., *Bull. Soc. Franc. Dermat. Syph.* 46:1076–1081, 1939.

POPOFF, L., *Dermat. Wehnschr.* 113:785–791, 1941.

POPOFF, L., and M. KUTINSCHEFF, *Dermat. Wehnschr.* 116:186, 1943.

POPOFF, L., In *Symposium Dermatologorum* (Prague, 1960), v. 1–3. Prague, Universita Karlova, 1962, v. 1, pp. 28–31; v. 3, pp. 27–30.

ROGERS, MALCOLM, M.D., "Can Doctors Distinguish Between Neurosis and Lupus Itself?", *Lupus News*, 1983.

ROGERS, MALCOLM, M.D., "Should You Seek a Second Medical Opinion?", *Lupus News*, 1984.

REYNOLDS, BARBARA JERRY, EMILY DICKINSON: A New Look at Her Life and Poetry Through Her Physical Illness, a Thesis Submitted in Partial Fulfillment of Requirement for a Degree of Master of Arts, University of Puget Sound, 1974.

REYNOLDS, JERRY FERRIS, "Banishment from Native Eyes": The Reason for Emily Dickinson's Seclusion Reconsidered by Jerry Ferris Reynolds, *The Markham Review*, published by the Horrmann Library of Wagner College.

11: A Personal Account of Living with Lupus

ALADJEM, HENRIETTA, *The Sun Is My Enemy*. New York: Prentice-Hall, 1972.

12: Lupus and Marriage

BLAU, SHELDON P., M.D. "Sex and Systemic Lupus Erythematosus," Brief Guide to Office Counseling, Arthritis Foundation, 1982.

13: Lupus and Pregnancy

BOYD, A., STODDAR, F. J., PIERCE, D. F.: Lupus erythematosus simulating toxemia of pregnancy. *Am. J. Obstet. & Gynec.* 74:1–62–1065, 1957.

CHETLIN, S. M., MEDSGER, T. A., JR., CARITAS, S. N.: Serum complement values during pregnancy in patients with systemic lupus erythematosus. *Arthritis Rheum.* 20:111, 1977.

CHETLIN, S. M., SHAPIRO, A. P., RODNAN, G. P., MEDSGER, T. A. JR., TOLCHIN, S. F., LEB., D. E., COHEN, P.: Plasma renin activity in progressive systemic sclerosis (scleroderma) with malignant hypertension. *Arthritis Rheum.* 20:111, 1977.

COX, J. B.: Disseminated lupus erythematosus in pregnancy. *Obstet. & Gynec.* 25:511–514, 1965.

DONALDSON, L. B., DE ALVAREZ, R. R.: Further observations on lupus erythematosus associated with pregnancy. *Am. J. Obstet. & Gynec.* 83:1461–1473, 1962.

FRIEDMAN, E. A., RUTHERFORD, J. W.: Pregnancy and Lupus Erythematosus. *Obstet. & Gynec.* 8:601, 1956.

HANSON, G. C., GHOSH, S.: Systemic lupus erythematosus and pregnancy. *B.M.J.* Nove. 1965, pp. 1227–1228.

McGee, C. D., Makowski, E. L.: Systemic lupus erythematosus in pregnancy. *Am. J. Obstet. & Gynec.* 107:1088–1012, 1970.

Morris, W. C.: Pregnancy in RA and SLE Aust. *NZI Obstet. Gynec.* 9:136–144, 1969.

Murd, A., Simpson, L., Rothfield, N. F.: Effect of pregnancy on course of SLE. *JAMA.* 183:917, 1963.

Van Kets, H. and Thiery, M.: Systemic lupus erythematosus and pregnancy. *Bull. Soc. Roy. Belg. Gynec. Obstet.* 37:469–476, 1967.

Wade, K.: Lupus erythematosus in pregnancy, *J. Arkansas Med. Soc.* 65:477–481, 1969.

Zurier, R. B., SLE & Pregnancy. *Clin. Rheum. Dis.* 1:613, 1975.

Zurier, R. B., Argyros, T. G., Urman, J. D., Warren, J. D., Rothfield, N. F.: SLE: Management During Pregnancy. *Obst. Gyn.* 51:178, 1980.

Glossary

ANTIBODY: Serum protein made in response to an antigen.

ANTIGEN: Protein that stimulates formation of antibodies.

ANTINUCLEAR ANTIBODY TEST: Blood test to detect antibodies to nuclei.

ARTHRALGIA: Aches and pains in one or many joints.

ARTHRITIS: Inflammation in a joint with heat, swelling, pain, and redness.

ASPIRIN: In 1763, researchers discovered that an extract of the willow bark was effective in relieving the pains of rheumatism. Willow extract owes its therapeutic efficacy to a substance called salicylic acid—from the Latin name for willow, *salix*. A chemically modified form, acetylsalicylic acid, is marketed under the name of aspirin. For reasons still unknown, aspirin helps relieve pain and reduce inflammation.

AUTOANTIBODY: Antibody directed against the body's own tissue.

AUTOGENOUS VACCINES: Vaccines made from the patient's own bacteria, as opposed to vaccines made from standard bacterial cultures.

AUTOIMMUNE: Sensitive to one's self; a person's body makes antibodies against some of its own cells.

BASAL METABOLISM TEST: Determines whether the body's metabolism is over- or underactive.

BASOPHIL: One of the granulated white blood cells.

BIOPSY: Sample of tissue taken for microscopic study.

BLOOD CELL: Three main kinds are recognized: red blood cells (erythrocytes) carry oxygen and carbon dioxide; white blood cells (leukocytes) help fight infection; platelets (thrombocytes) help prevent bleeding.

B LYMPHOCYTE (B CELL): Lymphocyte that makes antibodies.

BRONCHII: The tubes formed by the division of the windpipe, which convey air to the lung cells.

BUN: Blood urea nitrogen; when the kidneys fail, the BUN rises, as does the uric acid.

BUTTERFLY RASH: Form of double-wing-shaped skin rash around the nose and cheeks highly suggestive of lupus.

CAPILLARIES: Smallest of the blood vessels that connect arteries and veins.

CELL BIOLOGIST: One who studies cell architecture and function.

CHRONIC: Lasting for a long period of time.

CNS: Central nervous system.

COLLAGEN DISEASE: Group of diseases characterized by inflammation of connective tissues, especially the skin and joints—rheumatoid arthritis, SLE, scleroderma, Sjögren's syndrome, juvenile rheumatoid arthritis—also usually synonymous with rheumatic disease.

COMPLEMENT PROTEIN: Regulatory molecule of the immune response.

CONNECTIVE TISSUE: Substance that binds the body together, like a body glue. Connective tissue is the most widespread and abundant tissue in the body.

CORTICOSTEROID: Product of adrenal cortex.

CORTISONE: Pontent hormone of the adrenal glands; the pure compound was first discovered in adrenal secretion simultaneously in 1936 by Dr. Edward C. Kendall of the Mayo Clinic, and by Dr. Reichstein of Basel, Switzerland. It is now synthesized as a pure chemical.

COVALENT: Chemical bond formed by the sharing of electrons.

CUTANEOUS LESIONS: Visible changes in skin that are abnormal; rashes, sores, or scars.

CYTOPLASM: Part of the cell that surrounds its nucleus.

DEOXYRIBONUCLEIC ACID (DNA): Basic constituent of genes. Genes are the cellular constituents that govern heredity. Deoxyribonucleic acid is a large, complex molecule composed of chemicals called sugars and nucleic acids.

DERMATOMYOSITIS: A chronic inflammatory disease of the skin and muscles.

DIPLOPIA: Double vision.

DISCOID LUPUS: Lupus confined to the skin and characterized by atrophy and scarring.

DIURETIC: A drug that helps to make more urine.

DROPSY: Swelling of the legs and abdomen that is most often caused by heart failure, but can be due to kidney or liver disease.

EKG (OR ECG): Electrocardiogram, a recording of electrical forces from the heart.

ENDOCRINOLOGY: Study of the glands of internal secretion.

ENZYME: Protein substance that catalyzes a biological or chemical reaction.

ERYSIPELAS: Contagious, infectious disease of skin and subcutaneous tissue, marked by redness and swelling of affected areas and with constitutional symptoms.

ERYTHEMA NODOSUM: Painful red bumps on the skin; a skin manifestation of several diseases, but rarely of lupus.

ERYTHROCYTES: Normal nonnucleated red cells of the circulating blood; the red blood corpuscles.

ESTROGEN: Female hormone produced by the ovaries; it is responsible for secondary sexual characteristics in females and for the preparation of the uterus for implantation of the fertilized egg.

EXACERBATION: Recurrence of symptoms; another word for flare.

FALSE-POSITIVE SYPHILIS TEST: There are a number of tests for syphilis, including the Wasserman, RPR, Hinton, and VDRL tests. Some people will have a positive test for syphilis without having the disease. Systemic lupus erythematosus is one of the conditions that may give a positive test for syphilis, although syphilis is not present. This is called a false-positive test for syphilis. Lupus patients can make antibodies to a lipidlike (fatlike) substance structurally similar to the syphilis organism, and consequently may have a false-positive test for syphilis.

GALACTOSE: One of the sugars in milk, a part of the lactose molecule.

GASTRIC: Belonging to the stomach.

GASTRIC PARIETAL CELLS: Acid-producing cells of the stomach.

GENETIC: Pertaining to the genes; the word *genetic* refers to the property of transmission of parental characteristics to offspring. See DEOXYRIBONUCLEIC ACID.

GLOMERULONEPHRITIS: Type of kidney inflammation characterized by involvement of the glomerulus of the kidney.

HAPTEN: Chemical that will induce an immune response when coupled to a protein.

HEMATOLOGIST: Specialist in the study of blood.

HEMATURIA: Red blood cells in the urine.

HEMIPARESIS: Paralysis or weakness of one side of the body.

HEMOLYTIC ANEMIA: Condition characterized by a reduction in circulating red blood cells due to increased destruction of the cells by the body.

HEPATITIS: Inflammation of the liver.

HISTIOCYTE: Tissue macrophage—scavenger of cell debris, viruses, bacteria.

HISTOCOMPATIBILITY ANTIGEN (HLA): Cell-surface protein involved in transplant rejection; HLA proteins are controlled by genes on the sixth chromosome.

HISTOLOGY: Examination of tissue under a microscope as opposed to the gross clinical examination.

HISTOPATHOLOGY: Pathologic change in tissues and cells as seen under a microscope.

HLA SYSTEM: Genetic system controlling proteins on cell surfaces; often linked to disease.

HORMONE: From the Greek "to excite"; hormones are chemical messengers that excite a response in other tissue.

HYBRIDOMA: Fusion of an antibody-producing cell and a myeloma (tumor) cell that makes a great deal of monoclonal antibody.

HYDROXYCHLOROQUINE (PLAQUENIL): Antimalarial drug that has also been used as a treatment for lupus.

HYPERSENSITIVITY: Form of allergy generally mediated by antibodies.

HYPOCHONDRIAC: One who has morbid anxiety about health.

IMMUNE COMPLEXES: Specific combination of antibodies with their corresponding antigens.

IMMUNE MEDIATED: Produced by the immune system, i.e., antibodies and lymphocytes.

IMMUNE RESPONSE: Response of the body's immune system to antigens.

IMMUNITY: Power to resist infection.

IMMUNOFLUORESCENCE: Special technique of histology using a fluorescent dye to mark antibody or immune process taking place at a given site in the tissue.

IMMUNOGEN: Any substance capable of eliciting immunity.

IMMUNOLOGIC TOLERANCE: Specific suppression of immunity to antigens. Normally, we do not make antibodies to our own antigens, such as our own cells, tissue proteins, or DNA.

LE CELL TEST: The LE cell is a white blood cell that has eaten the nucleus of another white blood cell; the latter appears as a blue-staining spot inside the first cell.

LYMPHOKINE: Proteins made by monocytes and lymphocytes that affect other lymphocytes.

LYSE: To produce disintegration of cells, causing them to release their contents.

MACROPHAGES: Tissue cells that eat antigens, complexes, bacteria, and viruses.

MAJOR HISTOCOMPATIBILITY MARKER: See HISTOCOMPATIBILITY ANTIGEN.

MEPACRINE (QUINACRINE, ATABRINE): Antimalarial drug that was taken by U.S. Armed Forces personnel during World War II.

METABOLISM: Series of chemical processes in the living body by which life is maintained.

METHYLPREDNISOLONE: Synthetic form of corticosteroid.

MIXED CONNECTIVE TISSUE DISEASE: Consisting of two or more of the connective tissue diseases, e.g., lupus, polymyositis, scleroderma.

MOTOR APHASIA: Loss of speech due to a brain defect affecting the muscles of speech.

MUCOSAL IMMUNITY: Immunity of the gastrointestinal, genitourinary, or bronchial tracts.

MYASTHENIA GRAVIS: Disease in which nerve impulses are not properly transmitted to the muscle cells; as a result, muscles all over the body become weak.

NAPROXEN (NAPROSYN): One of several nonsteroidal antiinflammatory drugs (NSAIDs).

NATURAL KILLER CELL: Cell that kills (lyses) other cells.

NEPHRITIS: Inflamation of the kidney.

NEUROSIS: A disorder of the mental constitution.

NEUTROPHIL: Granulated white blood cell.

NICONACID: Swiss-French trademark for a preparation of nicotinic acid.

NICOTINAMIDE (NIACINAMIDE): Amide of 3-pyridinecarboxylic acid (niacin); its chemical formula is $C_6H_6N_2O$. A form of niacin.

NOXIOUS STIMULUS: Unpleasant or damaging substance or influence.

NUCLEOSIDE: One of the four types of building blocks of DNA.

NUCLEUS: That part of a cell containing DNA.

PANTOTHENIC ACID: Constituent of the vitamin B complex.

PATHOGENIC: Producing disease or undesirable symptoms.

PATHOLOGIST: Expert in pathology.

PATHOLOGY: Branch of medicine that deals with changes in tissues or organs of the body caused by or causing disease.

PELLAGRA: Deficiency of niacin (one of the B vitamins) that causes diarrhea, dermatitis, and demential (loss of intellectual function).

PENICILLIN: Any of a large group of antibiotics.

PERIARTERITIS NODOSA: Form of vasculitis (inflammation of blood vessels) affecting small and medium-sized blood vessels; may be caused by hepatitis.

PERIPHERAL NEUROPATHY: Malfunction of nerves of the arms or legs.

PERNICIOUS ANEMIA: Condition caused by vitamin B_{12} deficiency and characterized by a reduction in red blood cells and spinal cord abnormalities.

PHAGOCYTE: Cell (macrophage, monocyte) that ingests other cells or debris.

PHACOCYTOZED NUCLEAR MATERIAL: White cells that have ingested nuclei from other cells.

PHAGOCYTOSIS: Ingestion by phagocytes of foreign or other particles, or cells harmful to the body.

PHLEBITIS: Inflammation of a vein.

PHOTOSENSITIVITY: Sensitivity to light energy.

PLACEBO: Inactive substance given to a patient either for its pleasing effect or as a control in experiments with an active drug.

PLASMA: Fluid portion of the blood in which the blood cells float.

PLASMA CELL: Tissue cell that makes antibodies.

PLEURISY (PLEURITIS): Inflammation of the membrane between the chest wall and the lung.

POLYARTERITIS: Same as periarteritis nodosa.

POLYARTHRITIS: Inflammation of several joints at the same time.

POLYMORPHONUCLEAR LEUKOCYTE: Same as neutrophil.

PREDNISONE: Chemical name for a synthetic steroid hormone.

PROGESTERONE: Female hormone produced during pregnancy that is primarily responsible for maintaining pregnancy and developing the mammary glands.

PROPERDIN: One of the complement proteins.

PROSTAGLANDIN: The prostaglandins are a large family of pharmacologically active lipids (fats) widely distributed in mammalian tissue.

PROTEINS: Building blocks of the body; regulators of cell function.

PROTEINURIA: Protein in the urine.

PSYCHOSOMATIC: Relationship of the body to the mind; having bodily symptoms from mental rather than physical disorder.

PTOSIS: Drooping of an eyelid.

PULMONARY: Pertaining to the lungs.

PUPILLARY REACTION: Constriction or dilation of the pupil of the eye in response to light.

PURPURA: Rupture of blood vessels with leakage of blood into the tissues.

RENAL: Pertaining to the kidneys.

RHEUMATOID ARTHRITIS: Chronic inflammatory disease of the joints.

SCLERODERMA: "Hard skin," a chronic connective tissue disease characterized by leathery thickening of the skin; the internal organs may also be involved.

SEDIMENTATION: Settling of red blood cells to the lower portion of a volume of blood that has been treated to prevent clotting.

SERUM: Blood from which cells and fibrin have been removed.

SERUM CREATININE LEVELS: Creatinine is a substance normally found in blood in low concentration, since it is eliminated from the serum by the kidneys; high serum creatinine levels indicate malfunction of the kidneys.

SERUM PROTEIN: Any protein in the serum.

SIDE EFFECT: Adverse effect produced by a drug.

SJÖGREN'S SYNDROME: Autoimmune disease characterized by dryness of the mouth and eyes.

SPONTANEOUS REMISSION: Marked improvement in a disease that occurs without medical intervention.

STREPTOCOCCUS: Bacterium that may cause sore throats (strep throat) and skin infections (erysipelas, scarlet fever) that may result in nephritis, inflammation of the kidneys, or rheumatic fever (inflammation of the heart and joints).

SUBACUTE CUTANEOUS LUPUS ERYTHEMATOSUS: Lupus with characteristic skin lesions.

SULFADIAZINE: Antiinfective drug; one of the sulfonamides.

TESTIS: Synonym for testicle, the male reproductive organ responsible for production of sperm cells.

TETRACYCLINE: An antibiotic.

THERAPEUTICS: Study of the action of drugs and their application to the treatment of disease.

THERMAL BURNS: Injury to tissue caused by heat.

THROMBOCYTOPENIA: Reduction of circulating platelets.

THYROID GLAND: Gland located in the neck that produces thyroxine.

THYROIDITIS: Inflammation of the thyroid gland.

THYROXINE: Substance that affects the body's metabolic rate.

TITER: Highest dilution of a serum that gives a reaction with a substance.

T LYMPHOCYTE (T CELL): Lymphocyte involved in cellular immunity.

TOLERANCE TO NUCLEIC ACID ANTIGENS: Unresponsiveness to nucleic acids.

ULTRAVIOLET: Portion of the spectrum of sunlight that tans the skin.

UV-ALTERED DNA: DNA molecules disrupted by UV energy entering the cell, causing them to become antigen.

UV RADIATION: Radiation of energy of wavelengths 200 to 290 nm (UVC); 290 to 320 nm (UBV); 320 to 400 nm (UVA).

UREMIA: Marked kidney insufficiency characterized by nausea, vomiting, and even coma or convulsions, and a urine odor to the breath.

VASCULITIS: Inflammation of the blood vessels.

VASOMOTOR: Pertaining to control of the tone of the blood vessels; contraction of blood vessels causes blanching, whereas relaxation causes blushing.

VIRAL ETIOLOGY: Caused by a virus.

VIRAL PROTEIN: One of several constituents that make up a virus particle.

Index